Praise for

BioEnergetic Tools
for Wellness

"Dr. Lee Cowden is well-respected in the integrative medicine field, especially for bringing together successful treatment protocols for people with difficult health issues. In *BioEnergetic Tools for Wellness,* he and Connie Strasheim demonstrate the health benefits of using a wide variety of bioenergetic therapies that are effective for supporting the healing of common ailments. This is a great resource for people looking for solutions in bioenergetic medicine."

—Jane Oelke, ND, PhD
Natural Choices, Inc.

"For those faced with chronic illness, *BioEnergetic Tools for Wellness* provides an exceptional, first-hand look at bioenergetic healing technologies that have been proven to be successful for many, but which don't make the evening news. Whether you are a chronically ill patient seeking better solutions for wellness or a doctor looking for improved results in your patients, *BioEnergetic Tools for Wellness* should be your next resource to consult, as it will provide you with new options in the journey to wellness."

—Toby Watkinson, DC
Tobin Institute, Inc.

"*BioEnergetic Tools for Wellness* by Dr. Lee Cowden and Connie Strasheim is on the forefront of futuristic medicine. Energy/vibrational medicine is becoming the medicine of the future and this book clearly defines the tools that practitioners and patients can utilize to get well faster. It's a must-read because bioenergetic medicine will be at the cutting edge of the upcoming paradigm shift in effective and cost-efficient healthcare."

—Stephen T. Sinatra, M.D., F.A.C.C., F.A.C.N.
HeartMDInstitute.com

ACIM

The Journey to Wellness Book Series

BioEnergetic Tools for Wellness

How to Heal from Fatigue, Pain, Insomnia, Depression and Anxiety

W. Lee Cowden, MD, MD(H)
Connie Strasheim

ACIM Press

Books may be purchased in bulk by contacting
ACIMConnect.com, or Connie Strasheim at: Connie@ConnieStrasheim.com.

Cover Design: Nick Zelinger, NZ Graphics
Interior Design: Rebecca Finkel, F + P Graphic Design
Publisher: ACIM Press
Editor: John Maling, Editing By John
Publishing Consultant: Judith Briles, The Book Shepherd

First edition
Library of Congress Catalog Number: on file
ISBN paperback: 978-0-9961004-4-1
eISBN: 978-0-9961004-5-8

10 9 8 7 6 5 4 3 2 1

First Edition printed in USA, September, 2014

1. Health   2. Medicine   3. Wellness   4. BioEnergentic

Printed in the USA

Contents

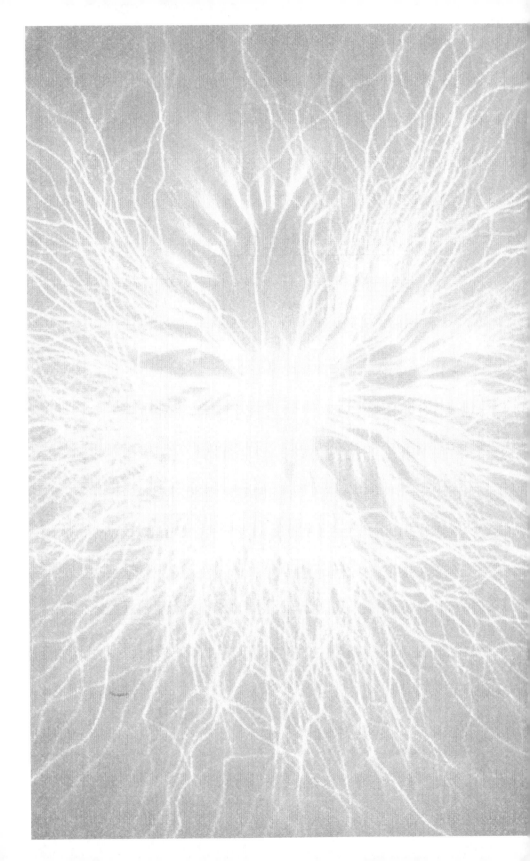

Foreword

Your body was designed to be healthy. It is not just a bag of bones or a bag of chemicals but a very sophisticated bioenergetic instrument that responds to outside electromagnetic influences— whether from the environment or the powerful tools found in bioenergetic medicine. If you take care of your body, utilize the right bioenergetic wellness tools, and avoid the chemical and electromagnetic toxins that you were never designed to be exposed to in the first place, then your body will usually move towards health and away from disease.

Sadly, this is not the perception of most Americans. They have been firmly led to believe that most disease and symptoms require the use of a prescription medication. The average adult is filling eleven prescriptions per year but after age 65 that increases to 31. This surprising number does not take into account any over-the-counter medications that are consumed.

Not only do these medications fail to address the cause of disease, but they also contribute to premature death and disability.

Estimates vary widely, but conservatively, over half a million preventable drug reactions occur every year in the United States alone. Even worse, over 100,000 people die needlessly every year from these drug reactions.

While the conventional medical model works exceptionally well for acute traumas, it fails miserably for virtually every other health challenge. The total number of premature unnecessary deaths attributable to the so-called health care system is well over 750,000 per year, leading many to believe that the conventional medical model, not heart disease or cancer, is the leading killer of Americans.

THERE IS GOOD NEWS!

While the above statistics can be disheartening, they are only shared to motivate you to action. You and your family never have to be one of these casualties. There are simple steps you can take that will put your body on a path toward healing and away from just about any disease you may ever encounter. Several of these steps are described in this book, as well as in the other books in Dr. Lee Cowden and Connie Strashiem's *Journey To Wellness* series.

Thankfully, the steps are really quite simple. I've studied medicine for over thirty years and the more I study, the clearer it becomes that health really is quite simple. Like any sport or complex endeavor, it nearly always boils down to following the basics.

Don't try anything fancy until you have mastered the basics, because for the vast majority of people, that is all that is needed. You typically won't need to purchase a shopping bag full of expensive supplements to regain your health; all you need to do is diligently apply the basics.

So, what are the basics?

I will list them in what I believe is their relative priority, so it is best to start from the top and work your way down. However, you don't have to master one before going on to the next. For many of you, these will be very basic steps but I can't emphasize enough how important integrating these basics into your life will be for you to recover or achieve optimal health.

Drink Enough Pure Water. There are two classes of chemicals in US tap water that can wreck your health. One is chlorine, which creates disinfection byproducts that are thousands of times more toxic than the chlorine itself. The other is fluoride, which has not been proven to have any beneficial effect on tooth decay when ingested, but has been shown to decrease IQ in children and increase the risk of thyroid disease.

Avoid Processed Foods. Over 95 percent of the food Americans eat is processed and loaded with chemicals, hormones and pesticides that will contribute to disease. More importantly, these foods are stripped of vital nutrients that your body needs to stay healthy. It is imperative you give your body the right fuel.

Pay Attention to the Timing of Your Meals. If you are one of the 85 percent of Americans that are overweight, have high blood pressure, diabetes or abnormal cholesterol levels, then you likely have insulin and/or leptin resistance. Our ancient ancestors never had access to a grocery store 24/7 and never consistently ate three meals a day.

Your genes and biochemistry aren't optimized for this eating pattern and when you are in constant feast mode you can easily accelerate disease. Restricting all the food you eat to an eight-hour window every day can help you to resolve insulin/leptin resistance. This is also called intermittent fasting, and is one of the most powerful dietary tools that I know of for accelerating your progress towards health. Time-restricting your eating is best done by skipping breakfast and then not eating for three hours before bedtime. This only needs to be done until your insulin and/or leptin resistance resolves.

Exercise Appropriately. We were designed to move frequently throughout the day and unfortunately, most of us simply don't exercise enough. Those of us that do are often wasting our time on cardio and aerobics. New research shows very clearly that exercise density is crucial for success. It is far better to do a few high intensity exercise sessions a week than spend monotonous hours on the treadmill. I call these high intensity exercises peak fitness. This should be balanced with strength training and stretching.

Get Outdoors and Enjoy the Sun. Science has now clearly shown that sensible exposure to the sun is necessary and should not be completely avoided, as many doctors recommend. One of its major benefits is that it enables your body to produce vitamin D if you expose enough of your skin to it during the right season. Vitamin D obtained from sun is far superior to the vitamin D in any oral supplement that you swallow, and you will never overdose on vitamin D from sunshine.

Be Sure to Get Enough Sleep. Most of us are only sleeping about six hours per night. This simply is not enough, as 7-8 hours nightly is what's typically required to repair and regenerate our bodies. It is important to make sure you sleep in complete darkness, and do not have any electrical or wireless devices nearby that can interfere with your sleep.

THE NEXT STEP IF THE BASICS FAIL TO RECOVER YOUR HEALTH

After practicing medicine for nearly thirty years and treating 25,000 patients, it is very clear to me that conventional medicine is focused primarily upon the chemical model of wellness. What I have found in my practice, however, is that the energetic model is a very helpful strategy for solving the health puzzle.

There are a wide variety of bioenergetic medicine clinicians out there but Dr. Cowden is one of the best that I know. I have known Lee for over 15 years and been very impressed with his depth of knowledge, compassion and ability to help seriously ill patients recover.

This book that he and Connie Strasheim have written is a great primer on bioenergetic medicine and testing. If you have applied the above-mentioned health principles and not yet recovered your health, it is my strong recommendation that you seriously consider a bioenergetic medical approach to help guide your next steps.

Dr. Lee Cowden is a USA board-certified cardiologist and internist who is internationally known for his knowledge and skill in practicing and teaching integrative medicine, and Connie Strasheim is a medical writer who has spent ten years recovering from Lyme disease and chronic fatigue syndrome using many of the tools described in this book.

Bioenergetic medicine is becoming more widely known in the West and has been used for centuries in the East, and has proven to be highly effective for healing the body of a variety of chronic and acute health conditions.

This book is a tremendous resource to assist you on your journey in moving away from symptomatic Band-Aids in the form of prescription drugs or surgery in order to find true healing.

In addition to a healthy diet, exercise and rest, the bioenergetic principles that Dr. Lee Cowden and Connie Strasheim share in this book can become a vital aspect of your daily regimen to help you bring your body towards balance so that you can take control of your health and experience healing from whatever health conditions that you may have.

—Joe Mercola, DO

Founder of Mercola.com, the world's most visited natural health site

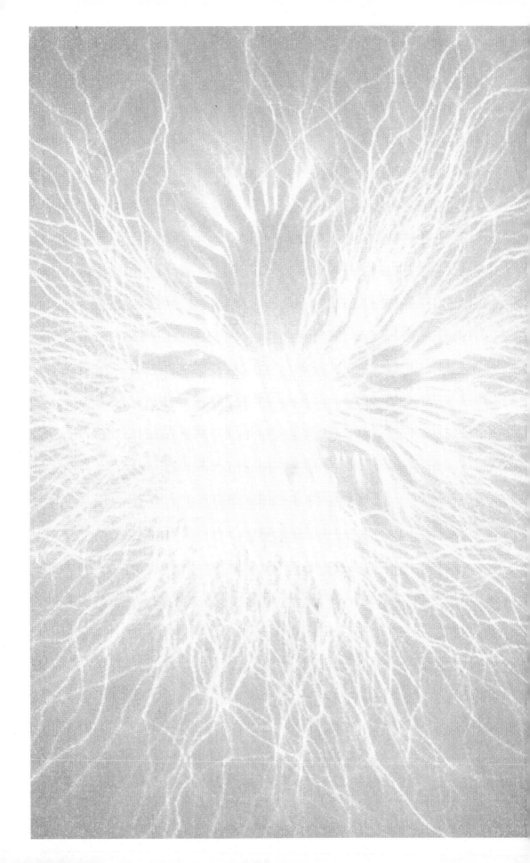

Part One
Wellness and BioEnergetic Balancing

CHAPTER ONE

Katherine's Story

Katherine sat in the waiting room of the lab, her stomach rumbling and palms sweaty. How many more of these fasting blood tests would she have to do before the doctors figured out what was wrong with her? Seems like she'd been here five or six times already over the past several months.

Yet her wise doctor finally believed he had discovered the cause of her woes—chronic Lyme disease. But would this test give him the answers he needed? After all, she had researched on Internet forums and recently discovered that even the best of lab tests were often inaccurate for diagnosing Lyme disease, because the infections suppressed the body's production of antibodies, and the microbes were experts at cloaking themselves and hiding from the immune system.

She sighed and checked her watch. Already she'd been in the waiting room thirty minutes. How long before she'd have to grab a granola bar to curb her crashing blood sugar? She pushed away thoughts of a hot cup of coffee and bowl of oatmeal. She needed to hang in there until her blood was drawn once again.

It was always the same. By the time she made it out of bed, took a shower, drove to the lab, waited for the blood draw, and came back home again, two hours would have usually passed—too long for a person with unstable blood sugar and weak adrenal glands.

More worries filled her mind. What if the test results were negative? Should she assume then that she didn't have Lyme disease? If not, then why did her limbs ache and why was she so tired? After all these tests, the doctors still didn't know....

Her friend Dana had recommended that she do a bioenergetic scan. Dana's doctor used a ZYTO device to detect problems in the body. The ZYTO, Dana claimed, could test for literally hundreds of infections, imbalances, and other problems that Katherine might have, in less than 30 minutes—and she wouldn't even have to fast or get poked with a needle. She would only have to place her hand atop a cradle while a computer scanned her body.

Still, Katherine wasn't sure. How could a device that "read" her body's energy field tell her whether she had Lyme disease? Yet these regular trips to the lab were getting old....

Katherine's frustrations may not seem like a big deal to you, unless you have struggled with chronic health challenges as she has, or known the frustration of having to do multiple tests for months, or years, without getting the answers that you need.

Even if you can't relate to her story, you can probably relate to not being able to discover the cause of some nagging symptom that you have because no conventional test or doctor has been able to tell you what it is. Or maybe you just wish that your doctor had better tests, besides those in conventional medicine, to help you determine what you need to do to be in optimal health.

Fortunately, bioenergetic medicine has some fantastic technologies and techniques for identifying problems in the body, as well as ways to remedy those problems, when conventional medicine or biochemical medicine cannot. With bioenergetic medicine, you can discover things about your health that no doctor or lab test can tell you.

In this book, we describe bioenergetic tools and evaluative techniques that are effective for remedying a multitude of health conditions. You don't have to be like Katherine—doing test after test trying to figure out what's wrong with you. One simple bioenergetic test can often tell you more about your health than twenty blood or urine tests. Similarly, bioenergetic medicine provides wellness solutions to augment the effectiveness of any biochemical treatments that your doctor might be giving you and, in some cases, can even replace them.

CHAPTER TWO

About BioEnergetic Medicine

We live in a fast-paced world, awash with environmental toxins, nutrient-deficient food, chronic illness, and difficult relationships. Many of us today feel sluggish or downright tired, or are depressed and irritable, or suffer from aches and pains that we can't seem to get rid of, no matter what we do. Even if we are in decent health, we might feel that we are operating at half-throttle at times, as the effects of our environment—from our relationships to the foods we eat—weigh upon our bodies, souls and spirits.

Despite our challenging environment, we believe that it's possible to prosper and be in excellent health if we are empowered with the right tools. We can have strong, balanced bodies, a peaceful, joyful and positive mindset, and a prosperous and productive life, if we are equipped with the right information, motivation, and willingness to step out and do what it takes to be well.

In this *Journey to Wellness* book series, we provide some fundamental tools for emotional, physical and spiritual well-being, which will help you to maintain, or attain wellness, whatever your current health condition.

Indeed, where conventional medicine has proven to be inadequate for diagnosing and healing the body, bio-energetic medicine has filled in the gaps, and gone beyond the limitations of allopathic (conventional) medicine strategies that are practiced in most hospitals and clinics in the United States and other "developed" nations.

In the first two books in the series, *Create a Toxin-Free Body & Home … Starting Today* and *Foods that Fit a Unique You,* we describe how eating the right foods for your unique biochemistry, and eliminating toxins from your body and home, can go a long way toward helping you to feel great and attain a superior level of wellness. No matter how you feel right now, if you do the things that we recommend in these books, you are likely to experience a higher level of well-being and feel better than you ever have before.

In this book, we discuss another powerful wellness tool that can take you to the next level in your healing journey—bioenergetic balancing, which is an essential adjunct to a proper diet, detoxification, and other tools that we describe in this series.

For the purposes of this book, we use the term "bioenergetic balancing" to refer to the concept of aligning or balancing the body's energy field to attain wellness. We use the term "bioenergetic medicine" to refer to specific healing tools that utilize the energy of devices, remedies, and the human body to achieve this balance.

Bioenergetic balancing can help your body to heal from a multitude of conditions. For the purposes of this book, we focus on its usefulness for eliminating fatigue, pain, insomnia, depression and anxiety—five conditions that most of us have suffered from at one time or another, or which you may currently be struggling with. In the following pages, we describe some excellent energy-balancing strategies for healing from these conditions, no matter their initial cause.

Even if you don't suffer from fatigue, pain, insomnia, depression or anxiety, you may find the information helpful for improving your current state of wellness, since the healing tools that we describe are useful for correcting many problems in the body—big or small.

Who among us wouldn't like to have a little more energy or vitality, or sleep a little better, or experience more positive emotions? The great thing about bioenergetic balancing is that it can be used as a tool to maintain your health as much as a tool to enhance it.

If you picked up this book, it's because you might know that bioenergetic medicine provides some amazing tools for wellness. Or maybe you don't know, but you are curious about what it has to offer. Maybe you have a friend or family member who was healed of an illness or health problem with bioenergetic wellness strategies, and now you want to know more.

Maybe you have nagging health problems, or even a severe illness, or you just want to learn about the different ways that bioenergetic balancing can help a friend or family member to feel better. If so, this book is for you!

Bioenergetic medicine is a broad term, encompassing possibly hundreds of types of wellness care modalities. For the purposes of this book, we share only those that we have personally found to be effective for eliminating symptoms of the aforementioned conditions (as well as many others).

These wellness care modalities range from electronic devices, to hands-on healing techniques, computerized testing devices and homeopathic remedies. We also describe the tools that we have found to be beneficial for assisting in the diagnosis of conditions that conventional (allopathic) medicine often misses.

Indeed, where conventional medicine has proven to be inadequate for diagnosing and healing the body, bioenergetic medicine has filled in the gaps, and gone beyond the limitations of allopathic medicine strategies that are practiced in most hospitals and clinics in the United States and other "developed" nations.

For that reason, we invite you to try out some of the diagnostic tools and healing strategies that are found within this book to see if they don't make you feel better—and take you to a whole new level of wellness!

We believe these remedies and strategies will improve your energy, vitality, mood, and quality of sleep, as well as other aspects of your well-being, and possibly bring you to a whole new level of health that you have never experienced before.

CHAPTER THREE

Why BioEnergetic Medicine?

Bioenergetics is becoming a buzzword in medicine today, especially in alternative and integrative medicine circles. While the East (Asia) has relied upon bioenergetic medicine for centuries, the West (North America and Europe) has only recently begun to understand its potential, power and effectiveness for healing the body from a multitude of conditions.

> Perhaps the most compelling reason to consider bioenergetic medicine is the simple fact that we are comprised of energy! Our bodies are not just bags of chemicals, but rather, very sophisticated electromagnetic instruments.

Most of us in the West have typically relied upon chemical substances to treat disease and imbalance in our bodies. For instance, we've been conditioned to take drugs for infections and pain medications or topical pain gels to treat pain. Few of us have probably used bioenergetic medicine, or energetic balancing, as a primary alternative to the chemical substances that we rely upon for symptom relief.

That said, you've likely been exposed to bioenergetic medicine in one form or another. For instance, if you have had pain, your doctor might have prescribed you TENS therapy or acupuncture. If you have had a viral infection, your naturopathic doctor might have given you a homeopathic remedy. Still, most of us in the West view bioenergetic medicine as an adjunct treatment for wellness—secondary in importance to supposedly more powerful or effective chemical treatments.

Other cultures, especially those in the East, such as the Chinese, utilize bioenergetic medicine as a primary healing modality, and they have often obtained better results in healing people of chronic diseases than those of us in the West.

Fortunately, in recent years, bioenergetic healing modalities have been exploding in the West amongst the integrative medical community, and their uses are expanding within conventional medicine. With the increased interest in this type of medicine, many kinds of bioenergetic treatments have become available, but we have found some to be more helpful than others for addressing problems in the body.

Bioenergetic medicine often provides a gentler and more effective alternative to the chemical treatments that are predominantly used in Western medicine. If you use the right therapy or treatment, you can often experience more powerful healing effects from a bioenergetic treatment than from a chemical one. Pharmaceutical drugs and other conventional therapies often fail to make us well. So here we suggest powerful, proven effective bioenergetic strategies that can help you to heal from a variety of common health conditions.

We encourage you to consider bioenergetic medicine as a primary wellness tool that can enhance your physical, mental, emotional and spiritual well-being as much as a healthy diet, exercise or rest. Consider it an important component of your daily regimen, to maintain and preserve good vitality or to help bring your body into better balance.

Perhaps the most compelling reason to consider bioenergetic medicine is the simple fact that we are comprised of energy! Our bodies aren't just bags of chemicals, but rather, very sophisticated electromagnetic instruments. The energy of our bodies is measurable. And did you know that when a biochemical change occurs in your body, it is commonly preceded by a bioenergetic change?

Some people associate bioenergetic medicine with divine spiritual energy work. For the purpose of this book, we will be describing strategies that balance the body's physiological and electromagnetic energy systems through physical and/or quantum physical means, rather than with spiritual energies.

Energy healing can also refer to, and come from, super-natural or divine energy, but we believe that the body's innate energy and divine energy are different. That is, the measurable electromagnetic energy of the body isn't the same energy that comes from the spiritual realm.

Some practitioners draw upon energy from the spiritual realm to enhance the effects of therapies that balance the body's natural electromagnetic energy, but we believe that this can be a potentially dangerous practice—and is best avoided. We have found that some practitioners, even well intentioned ones, can unwittingly invite harmful spiritual energy into their work. So unless you truly understand the source of the energy, it is best to only work with the body's innate electromagnetic field.

Bioenergetics is becoming a buzzword in medicine today, especially in alternative and integrative medicine circles. While the East has relied upon bioenergetic medicine for centuries, the West has only recently begun to understand its potential power and effectiveness for healing the body from a multitude of conditions.

Regardless of your spiritual beliefs, bioenergetic healing techniques that draw upon the energy of your body's own electromagnetic field or which come from bioenergetic devices or remedies can be profoundly healing.

CHAPTER FOUR

Proof that We Are Energetic Beings

Your body's energy is both electrical and magnetic, which is why it is referred to as "electromagnetic." And indeed, modern medical tests have proven that our bodies have both electricity and magnetism.

Conventional (or allopathic) medicine has often tried to prove that bioenergetic medicine is quackery, but if the body is comprised of energy, and this energy is quantifiable and measurable, then why couldn't outside sources of energy influence it, for better or for worse?

The electrocardiogram, for instance, displays electrical impulses that come from the heart. This electricity regulates the contraction and pumping of blood from the heart to the organs and muscles. The magneto-cardiogram shows that same process magnetically.

Then there's the electroencephalogram, which displays electrical activity from the brain, and the electromyogram, which measures electrical impulses from the skeletal muscles. In addition, doctors do nerve conduction velocity studies that show electrical currents within nerve pathways.

Every cell in your body produces some electricity and some magnetism. Some types of cells produce high amounts of electricity and magnetism that can be easily measured with medical equipment. Heart cells are one such type. Other types of cells make less energy; however, this energy can still be detected with sensitive medical instruments.

Conventional (allopathic) medicine has often tried to prove that bioenergetic medicine is quackery, but if the body is comprised of energy, and this energy is quantifiable and measurable, then why couldn't outside sources of energy influence it, for better or for worse?

For every electrical event that occurs in the body, there is also a corresponding magnetic event. So every time your body produces an electrical signal, it also produces a magnetic field, which can be measured with medical instruments. For instance, as we mentioned above, a magnetocardiogram measures the magnetic field produced by your heart.

Similarly, in our environment, wherever there is an electrical field, there is also a magnetic field. This is why the energy from cell phones, microwave towers, household wiring, appliances and the like are referred to as electromagnetic radiation (EMR). An excess of this radiation is referred to as electromagnetic pollution.

Whenever you expose your body to an electromagnetic field (EMF), for example, that which comes from poor household wiring, or a nearby cell phone tower, your body gets continually bombarded with electrical EMF pulses. The magnitude of those pulses can disrupt the normal functioning of your cells' energy. We describe more about the harmful effects of EMFs in the next chapter.

Energy isn't static, but rather, a dynamic phenomenon, continually moving and flowing. The lights in your home, for instance, get switched on because of conduction electrons—"loose" packets of energy—that can move within and along the electrical wires forming a conduction path, extending from the power station to your house and back. The loose, metal-wire electrons—conduction electrons—actually jiggle back and forth due to the AC (alternating current) voltages generated by the power station within the power lines.

When you turn on the lights in your house, the jiggling electrons lose a bit of energy to the filaments of the light bulbs because their resistance is higher than that of the electrical wire, and they convert that energy into heat and light radiation. The excess energy that wasn't needed to turn on and create that heat and light is still available along the conduction path and is sent back to the power station, ready to be re-circulated through the power lines and converted into other forms of energy.

Similarly, energy continually moves throughout your body, causing certain biochemical events to occur in synchronicity. For instance, electrons move continually throughout your nervous system, in a "depolarization" wave (this occurs when an electrical charge builds up and then dissipates as the physical or chemical reaction that it drives goes forward), every time you have a thought, contract a muscle, or experience pain. Every action of your body—physical or chemical—requires energy.

The Chinese might have been the first to observe how energy moves throughout the human body. They discovered the acupuncture meridian system more than 2000 years ago, which details specific pathways and points along the body through which "Qi" or life energy flows. Through empiric observation, they noted that energy flows in an orderly fashion along these pathways.

Then, in the 1950s, a German medical doctor and engineer, Dr. Reinhard Voll, as well as other researchers, started using instruments to measure electrical conductance at various acupuncture points on the skin. They discovered that the movement of electrons through the skin at acupuncture points was 20 to 50 times greater than on other points on the skin that were just a quarter of an inch away.

Dr. Voll verified through these tests that the hundreds of acupuncture points that the Chinese had discovered and described over 2000 years ago were exactly where they had said they were on the body. Dr. Voll thus proved through scientific instrumentation that the Chinese observations were correct.

Some two decades later, in the 1970s, French researcher, Pierre de Vernejoul, injected radioactive isotopes into acupuncture points on a group of patients, and, through nuclear imaging, discovered that the nuclear radioactive isotopes didn't distribute uniformly throughout their bodies, but instead traveled quickly up the meridians that the Chinese had discovered twenty centuries before! So the French also proved, through their testing, the existence of energy meridians, albeit it a mere two millennia later!

Anatomists have also discovered that there are more papillae (small, nipple-like projections on the surface of the skin) at acupuncture points than on other parts of the skin, even those just a quarter of an inch away. These papillae have blood vessels and nerves that project upwards from the lower layers of the skin to the epidermis, which could explain why there is greater electrical conductance at those points.

And recently, Zang-Hee Cho, a University of California Irvine professor, proved with functional MRI brain scanning that when you stick a needle in the "eye point" on the little toe, the same area of the brain is stimulated as when you directly stimulate the eye itself with a needle. This experiment further proves the existence of energy pathways in the body.

The acupuncture meridian system is still a mystery to researchers, as it doesn't correlate with any physical structure in the body. The meridians are not nerves, but there is something in the body that moves energy along those pathways.

CHAPTER FIVE

Where Our Energy Comes From and How We Use It

So where does our energy come from? Well, the body doesn't synthesize energy from nothing; it takes substances with energy in them—such as food—and extracts energy from them.

It all starts with the sun. Plants receive energy from the sun in the form of light photons (packets of light energy), and then synthesize various substances from that light radiation energy. They do this with the aid of chlorophyll, a complex chemical molecule inside the plant leaf that is similar in structure to the hemoglobin that is found in our red blood cells.

> This energy is used by the cell for a variety of functions, including synthesizing proteins and other chemicals as well as for transporting nutrients into our cells and toxins out of them. Energy is necessary and vital for our cells to work properly.

Chlorophyll absorbs sunlight, which results in in the production of electrons that ultimately are used to convert atmospheric carbon dioxide into carbohydrates and other nutrients. When we eat leaves from a plant containing these carbohydrates, our bodies break down the carbohydrates into sugars that are absorbed into our bloodstream as nutrients for our cells. The sugars are carried by our bloodstream throughout our body to our cells, which exert other chemical actions upon the sugars in order to extract the energy from them.

Electromagnetic pollution, for instance, can be a primary or contributing cause to a multitude of chronic degenerative diseases. Electromagnetic pollution comes from sources such as wireless technology, power lines, smart meters, poor wiring in the home, appliances and microwave towers.

Just as energy is responsible for carrying out the functions of our bodies on a macro level, so it is also primary in the functioning of our bodies on a micro level. For instance, the mitochondria, which is an organelle (a complex structure) inside our cells that metabolizes sugars and fats to create energy, is where most of our cellular energy—approximately 95 percent— is manufactured.

This energy is used by the cell for a variety of functions, including synthesizing proteins and other chemicals as well as for transporting nutrients into our cells and toxins out of them. Energy is vital for our cells to work properly.

Cell membranes, or the outer coverings of cells, also have energy, and the difference in electrical potential between the interior and exterior of the cell is referred to as the electrical transmembrane potential. The transmembrane potential, or stored energy within the cell membrane, determines how effective our cells are at fulfilling different functions, such as carrying signals along nerve or brain cells, or contracting heart muscle cells.

When our cell membranes leak, due to electromagnetic pollution and other types of contamination, then their electrical potential across the cell membrane decreases, and the cells become less effective at carrying out their activities.

For instance, if your brain cells are mildly affected by electromagnetic pollution on a regular basis, you might become forgetful. Or if they are severely affected, you might have seizures. If your heart cells are affected, you might have life-threatening arrhythmias or develop an irregular heartbeat.

A healthy person might have a transmembrane potential of -70 millivolts, but if that membrane is disrupted by electromagnetic pollution, for instance, that number might be reduced to -30 or -40 millivolts. When the transmembrane potential gets this low, it can result in a myriad of health problems such as arrhythmias and other heart conditions; seizures, muscle twitches and other musculoskeletal problems; Leaky Gut syndrome (a condition whereby undigested food particles pass through the intestinal wall and cause inflammation); cancer and chronic fatigue, just to name a few!

This is why keeping your transmembrane potential high with bioenergetic balancing and other wellness strategies and maintaining the energy of your cells at a proper level is so essential for good health.

CHAPTER SIX

Electromagnetic Pollution

Just as the right type of energy can be used to heal the body, so can the wrong type of energy damage or destroy it.

Electromagnetic pollution, for instance, can be a primary or contributing cause to a multitude of chronic degenerative diseases. Electromagnetic pollution comes from sources such as wireless technology, power lines, smart meters, poor wiring in the home, appliances and microwave towers.

> **Many studies that link EMF exposure to cancer and other diseases can be found in the BioInitiative Report (*BioInitiative.org*), a compilation by 29 independent scientists and health experts from around the world.**

Our energy is disrupted when we are exposed to environmental electro-pollution. When this happens, our cells can't effectively remove waste, receive nutrients or carry out any of the other functions that are necessary for maintaining life. They also leak out nutrients, especially potassium and magnesium, which are essential for proper cellular function.

Scientific studies have also proven that electromagnetic frequencies (EMFs) damage DNA by generating free radicals and creating cell mutations that lead to cancer. Certain types of cancer, including brain cancer and acoustic neuroma, (cancer of the inner ear) are directly caused by electromagnetic fields from cell phones. These fields disrupt the cell's transmembrane potential, resulting in acid buildup inside the cell and changes in the cell's metabolism that lead to cancer. And if the electrical potential of a cell gets low enough, it can become spontaneously cancerous.

Electromagnetic pollution also alters your body's ability to manufacture neurotransmitters and hormones, which play an integral role in the functioning of your immune system. It disrupts the normal functioning of your neurological, cardio-vascular, and endocrine (hormone) systems, by altering inter- and intracellular communication. It disrupts your blood-brain barrier, which separates the blood from the brain's extracellular fluid in the central nervous system. This barrier helps to keep toxins out of your brain, and nutrients in.

Many studies that link EMF exposure to cancer and other diseases can be found in the BioInitiative Report *(BioInitiative.org)*, which is compiled by 29 independent scientists and health experts from around the world.

Fortunately, a number of bioenergetic healing modalities, some of which we will be describing in this book, can restore normal energy and proper function to the cells when they have been damaged by dangerous electromagnetic fields from the environment.

It used to be that if you wanted to be healthy, all you had to do was eat your veggies, exercise and get good sleep—but not anymore! The amount of pollution to which we are all exposed, including EMF pollution, has meant that we also must do things to protect ourselves from its effects upon our bodies.

For instance, unless you live out in the country, it's a good idea to sleep under a Faraday cage at night, which is a protective, silver-lined mesh canopy net that blocks out high-frequency electromagnetic fields. If you are continually exposed to high levels of EMFs while you sleep, you can't effectively regenerate your body at night,

Other things that you can do to reduce your exposure to EMFs include: unplugging all of the appliances in your bedroom at night and/or turning off the circuit breakers in your home which supply power to your bedroom area, and painting your walls with EMF shielding paint.

Measuring EMFs

You can get a general idea about the amount of low-frequency EMFs that you are exposed to in your home by purchasing a $35 Gauss meter on the Internet.

Low-frequency EMFs most often come from sources such as household appliances, wall wiring and power lines. The higher frequencies, which come from cell phone and microwave towers, wireless technology, smart meters and baby monitors, must be measured with a higher frequency meter, such as a Trifield 100XE meter, which costs about $120 to $250. However, these meters only measure frequencies up to 3 GHz.

To get an idea about the levels of high-frequency EMFs in your environment, it's better to purchase a device that can measure fields up to 8 GHz. The EMF Safety Store, *EmfSafetyStore.com*, sells all types of meters, including one that measures up to 8 GHz and which costs approximately $500. Purchasing a meter with several other people is one way to defray its expense.

It's a good idea to periodically reassess the EMFs in your environment, since new microwave towers, power lines, and other sources of EMFs are continually being constructed. Most of us are exposed to high levels of EMFs daily, so regardless of where you live, unless your home is out in the countryside, we recommend looking for ways to avoid or protect yourself from EMFs in order to optimize your health.

For a comprehensive explanation of EMFs, their dangers, how they affect your body, and what you can do to protect yourself against their effects, we encourage you to check out the first book in this series, *Create a Toxin-Free Body & Home ... Starting Today*. Electromagnetic pollution is a broad but important topic to understand in today's world, and we highly recommend that you read more about it so that you know how to keep your energy balanced and your body as healthy as possible.

CHAPTER SEVEN

Geopathic Stress

Geopathic stress is another source of energetic pollution in the environment that can also negatively affect our bodies' energy.

Some researchers suspect that geopathic stress is a common factor in many illnesses, including some cardiovascular conditions, attention deficit disorder (ADD), immune deficiency disorders and chronic fatigue syndrome.

Geopathic fields are lines or zones that run over the entire surface of the earth and emit electromagnetic energy. These zones are created by geological features, including faults in the earth, underground cavities, streams, metal veins and mineral concentrations. Underground cables, pipes, road construction projects and other man-made alterations of the earth can also create geopathic stress zones.

While geopathic stress is a relatively new concept in bioenergetic medicine, it was actually first discovered in the 1940s by the German researcher Baron von Pohl. Von Pohl noticed that people who slept on a geopathic field for an extended period of time often eventually developed cancer. He witnessed this phenomenon with several generations of people.

Dr. Cowden and other researchers have observed that cats prefer to sleep over areas of geopathic stress, while dogs avoid them!

Some researchers suspect that geopathic stress is a common factor in many illnesses, including some cardiovascular conditions, attention deficit disorder, immune deficiency disorders and chronic fatigue syndrome.

Signs and symptoms of exposure to geopathic or EMF stress include but are not limited to: chronic pain, fatigue, headaches, brain fog, irritability and insomnia. Both EMF and geopathic stress have also been linked to learning difficulties, behavioral problems and neurological disabilities in children. This has been proven in scientific studies, many of which you can find on the Bioinitiative Working Group website: *BioInitiative.org.*

Sleeping in a geopathic stress zone is particularly harmful, since the body repairs and regenerates itself at night, and this process becomes interrupted by the radiation from these zones.

Fortunately, these zones, which are found everywhere, are typically only five to six inches wide, so if you happen to be sitting or lying on one, it's not that difficult to move off or away from them. But how do you know if you are sitting or lying directly over a geopathic stress zone?

Unfortunately, geopathic fields can be difficult to measure with instruments. A device called a Geomagnetometer is useful for this purpose, but they are expensive—about $750 on the Internet. Therefore, it's best to hire a building biologist to do an inspection of your home, to help you identify the areas of geopathic stress.

Another way that you can potentially identify a geopathic field is to sleep on the other side of your bed. If you sleep better on one side of your bed than on the other, chances are there is a geopathic field on the side of your bed where you don't sleep well.

Building biologists can also measure the amount of electromagnetic radiation to which you are exposed, and make recommendations about how you can protect yourself from it. The International Institute for Building Biology and Ecology: *hbelc.org/findexpert/enviroconsult.html* contains a list of some building biologists in the US and around the world. This list is not comprehensive, and because building biology is a relatively new specialty in the United States, specialists may be difficult to find in some small towns and cities.

> In over 25 years of working with patients, I have observed that EMF and geopathic fields have a negative synergistic effect upon the body. If you are exposed to both at the same time, it can have a huge negative impact upon your health. Since we are all swimming in a sea of EMFs, it's a good idea to ensure that we aren't all sleeping over geopathic fields, too.
> —Dr. Lee Cowden

If you can't find a building biologist to help you identify the location of the geopathic fields in your home, there are a couple of other ways that you may be able to identify them.

First, if you have pets, they can help you to do this. Dr. Cowden and other researchers have observed that cats prefer to sleep over areas of geopathic stress, while dogs avoid them. So if you have a dog and cat at home (or your neighbor has a dog and cat that you can "borrow" for a few days), notice where they sleep on your bed. You'll then want to make sure to sleep where the dog sleeps, but not where the cat sleeps.

Babies also don't sleep well on geopathic fields. They will usually move off of them until they are about a year old. If you happen to have an infant that moves to a specific place on the bed at night, it may be because he or she is moving off of a stress zone.

While geopathic stress is a relatively new concept in bioenergetic medicine, it was actually first discovered in the 1940s by the German researcher Baron von Pohl. Von Pohl noticed that people who slept on a geopathic field for an extended period of time often eventually developed cancer.

Another way that you can potentially identify a geopathic field is to sleep on the other side of your bed. If you sleep better on one side of your bed than on the other, chances are there is a geopathic field on the side of your bed where you don't sleep well. Or, try moving your bed to the right or to the left a few feet, or elsewhere in your bedroom, to see if you feel any differently.

You may be unable to fall asleep or stay asleep, or you might awaken feeling un-refreshed, tired or with aches and pains if you are sleeping on a geopathic field. So if you sleep with a partner and one of you awakens feeling exhausted and terrible, but the other feels okay (and neither of you are aware of having a health problem), then the one who feels bad or unrested is likely to be sleeping on a geopathic field. To verify this, switch places with your partner for a few nights to see if either of you feels any differently.

OTHER FACTORS THAT CAUSE STAGNANT ENERGY AND BAD HEALTH IN YOUR BODY

Your energy can be disrupted by EMFs, but toxins and other factors can also cause it to stagnate or become unbalanced. If environmental toxins build up in your tissues and organs, for example, then you might develop symptoms or disease there. The Chinese learned this 2000 years ago when they discovered the acupuncture meridian system.

Keeping your energy balanced will enhance the beneficial effects of your diet, detoxification regimen, and anything else that you do for wellness.

Yet even seemingly less damaging things can obstruct your energy. Scars across your body's meridians, for instance, can disrupt energy flow, as can metal. Metal watches, belts, metallic jewelry, wire-rimmed glasses and underwire bras can disrupt the energy flow through acupuncture meridians much in the same way that a metal wrench causes a short circuit when it's accidentally dropped across two uninsulated wires in an attic.

In addition, metals on the body can act as antennas that pick up and amplify into the body the ambient electromagnetic radiation from Wi-Fi, cordless phones, cell phone towers, and other sources of electromagnetic energy. Therefore, it is best to avoid wearing metal, especially if you know that you are sensitive to the effects of EMFs.

> **Energetic testing can often "fill in the blanks" and provide information about our bodies that conventional tests miss.**

By now we hope you are convinced that there is ample evidence to prove that we are electromagnetic beings, and that our energy, and consequently, our biochemistry, can be influenced by outside sources of energy, for better or for worse!

If you want to increase the vitality and health of your body, it is a good idea to not only pay attention to your biochemistry—but also your energy! In reality it is a two-way street: our biochemistry is influenced by energy, and our energy is also influenced by our biochemistry.

For this reason, we recommend lifestyle and health maintenance practices that directly address both your biochemistry and your body's energy system.

For instance, in the first two books in this series, *Foods that Fit a Unique You* and *Create a Toxin-Free Body & Home...Starting Today,* we describe the importance of eating the right foods and removing physical toxins from your body with different therapies and toxin removal agents.

Maintaining a healthy diet and a clean body and home are two of the most important things that you can do to be well—but if you want to feel your best, we also recommend incorporating some bioenergetic balancing strategies into your daily or weekly routine. Keeping your energy balanced will enhance the beneficial effects of your diet, detoxification regimen, and anything else that you do for wellness.

Energy can hinder our well-being or promote it, depending upon whether we expose ourselves to harmful EMFs or harness the beneficial effects of bioenergetic medicine.

What's more, if you have a health condition or chronic illness, balancing your energy can enable your body to remove toxins more efficiently, and heal you, when drugs, herbs, supplements and other strategies fail to do so.

In the following chapters, we describe five common symptoms, or health conditions that most of us have suffered from at one time or another—and which can result from chronic illness, or simply the stresses of daily living. We then provide information on some of the best bioenergetic tools to help you to heal from these conditions, regardless of their cause.

CHAPTER EIGHT

Gary's Story

Gary tossed and turned beneath his comforter, but sleep would not come. He glanced at his alarm clock for the third time and heaved a sigh. He envisioned lugging his exhausted body to work after yet another sleepless night.

His doctor had written him a prescription for a sleep medication, since none of the natural remedies that his naturopathic doctor had given him were helping him to rest, but Gary cringed at the thought of becoming addicted to a drug. He had friends who had been prescribed antidepressants for sleep, and their insomnia only seemed to get worse.

Still, he had to rest. He didn't mind being a little tired—but his work as a CPA was intense and he couldn't afford to have his mind in a fog from lack of sleep.

He phoned his sister Stephanie who always was working on some bizarre art project until the wee hours of the morning. If only he were like his sister and could work and sleep whenever he felt like it!

She answered the phone and immediately chastised him. "Gary, what did I tell you about that smart meter? You were sleeping fine until they put that thing on your house! You need to get it removed … and turn off those circuit breakers at night. I'm telling you, those things are why you can't sleep."

Gary cringed. He was tired of his sister's off-the-wall health theories. He had never known anyone to have insomnia because of electromagnetic radiation. But now he was getting desperate, and almost willing to try anything just to get some shut-eye.

The next day, and feeling like a fool, he contacted the electric company and asked them to remove the smart meter. Fortunately, as Stephanie had told him, he would be able to get it removed, since the laws in California allowed its residents to choose whether or not they wanted to have smart meters on their homes. He also followed her instructions to unplug his alarm clock and turn off the circuit breakers in his bedroom at night.

Within a few days, Gary began sleeping soundly again. Oh, why hadn't he listened to his sister sooner? The past two years wouldn't have been such a nightmare …

As Gary's story illustrates, electromagnetic energy matters! It can hinder our well-being, or promote it, depending upon whether we expose ourselves to harmful EMFs or harness the beneficial effects of bioenergetic medicine.

CHAPTER NINE

Do-It-Yourself and Doctors' Diagnostic Techniques

Bioenergetic evaluative techniques and devices are great tools that can help you to diagnose disease, discern nutritional and other imbalances, and determine what your body needs at any given time. Muscle testing, electrodermal devices, Chinese pulse testing and thermography, among other testing modalities, are just a few ways to test your body for problems, using your body's own energy and/or that of a testing device.

There are some do-it-yourself muscle-testing techniques that you can learn on your own and which you can perform alone or with a partner (if you are ambitious and intuitive!). By learning these techniques, you can determine, from the comfort of your home, and without having to see a doctor or do a lab test—the types of foods and nutritional supplements that your body most needs, among other things.

Typically, whenever most of us have a health problem and need to find out what's wrong, or just want to know what our bodies need nutritionally, we go to a holistic or conventional medical doctor to have a blood, urine or saliva test done. Unfortunately, these tests, while essential, don't always provide the complete picture about what we need. Energetic testing can often "fill in the blanks" and provide information about our bodies that conventional tests miss.

We don't advocate not doing conventional tests in favor of doing energetic ones. Indeed, both types of testing are important, but we encourage you to work with a healthcare practitioner that does some type of energetic testing in conjunction with conventional blood, urine, stool, saliva or imaging tests. This will provide you with the most comprehensive picture about your health, and what you need to recover or simply feel your best.

In the following chapters, we describe a few of the most common and effective ways that you can test your body to find out what it needs, using bioenergetic devices and techniques. For most of these, you will need to work with a licensed health care practitioner who is skilled in their use.

However, in the next chapter, we also describe a technique called muscle testing that you can learn to do yourself, from the comfort of your home. Muscle testing can help you to determine the foods and supplemental nutrients that your body needs, among other things.

CHAPTER TEN

Muscle Testing

Muscle testing, of which there are many types, such as Contact Reflex Analysis (CRA) and Autonomic Response Testing (ART), utilizes your body's energetic field and muscle responses to identify potential health problems, as well as the remedies and foods that your body most needs to heal or remain well. It is used by many practitioners of alternative and integrative medicine, and is a powerful and effective evaluative tool, when you or the person who is doing the testing is skilled in its use.

Every skeletal muscle in your body is attached to or associated with your autonomic nervous system (ANS). The autonomic nervous system is mostly responsible for the automatic functions of the body, such as heart rate, digestion, respiration, perspiration, urination and blood pressure. If you do something that causes distress to your ANS, it will momentarily distress all of the muscles that are attached to your ANS.

If, for instance, you test a food that you are allergic to using muscle testing, your ANS will respond by causing the muscles of your body to become momentarily weak. But if you test a muscle, or group of muscles again after you remove the food from your body or energy field, then the muscle or muscles will become strong again.

A weak muscle response indicates that your body did not like whatever you were testing—whether that thing was a food, vitamin supplement or drug. Conversely, a strong muscle response indicates that your body would likely benefit from whatever you tested. The stronger the muscle response, the more your body would probably benefit from it.

As we already mentioned, there are a variety of types of muscle testing. And if you have a serious health condition, it's best to get a diagnosis about that condition from a health care practitioner who utilizes muscle testing, along with other tests, rather than try to test yourself using the techniques that we describe in this section.

However, there are some do-it-yourself muscle-testing techniques that you can learn on your own and which you can perform alone or with a partner (if you are ambitious and intuitive!). By learning these techniques, you can determine from the comfort of your home, and without having to see a doctor or do a lab test—the types of foods and nutritional supplements that your body most needs, among other things.

The basic techniques of muscle testing are easy to learn, but take some time to master, so don't give up if you don't get accurate results right away.

The first thing that you must do when muscle testing is determine whether you are "testable." Muscle testing will not work properly if your body's energy is too imbalanced or out of alignment. You can become temporarily un-testable and energetically imbalanced for many reasons. The most common of these include: if you are emotionally stressed or dehydrated, are standing over a geopathic field, or just ate a food or consumed a substance that you were allergic to.

Fortunately, there are ways that you can bring your energy into better balance so that you can obtain accurate results while muscle testing. We describe how in the following sections.

First, to determine whether you are testable, stand in front of a counter or table, close your eyes and place your left palm over your belly button, without allowing your left fingers to touch your abdomen. Leave your right hand down at your side. Wait for a moment and try to discern any slight movement of your body. You should either feel yourself leaning back onto your heels slightly, leaning forward, or not moving at all.

If you find yourself leaning backwards slightly, this means that you are "testable" and you should be able to reliably test yourself for different substances or foods. Once you have determined that you are testable, you don't want to move from your position, so make sure that the foods or remedies that you want to test are within arms' reach.

If, when you put your left palm over your belly button with your eyes closed, you either don't move or lean forward slightly, then it means that you are not likely to obtain accurate test results, either because you are standing over a geopathic field or are untestable for some other reason.

To find out whether you are standing on a geopathic field, move two or three feet away from the area where you were previously standing and test yourself again, with your eyes closed and left palm over your belly button. Try moving backward, forward, and to the left and/or right a couple of feet, until you get a better response.

If your body responds differently than before, and becomes testable, then it probably means that you were previously standing on a geopathic field and should not remain there when testing yourself in the future. If changing your position doesn't change the outcome of your test results, then something else may be blocking your energy and causing you to be untestable.

For instance, you may be blocked due to emotional stress. If you are under a lot of stress, you can try unblocking yourself by placing the palm of your right hand over your forehead and your left palm over your belly button while doing the standing test with your eyes closed. By keeping your right palm on your forehead during testing, you can remove the influence of any emotional stress upon your body.

Or, if you think that you have just eaten an allergenic or toxic food, this too can affect your ability to obtain accurate test results, so it is best to test yourself several hours after eating. To reverse the energy-blocking effects of allergenic and toxic foods, hold your right index fingertip about an inch above the bottom end of your sternum (the breast bone in the midline of your chest), during the muscle testing process to see if that unblocks the energy flow. If so, keep your right index fingertip on that sternum point throughout the testing process.

You can also use a universally allergenic or toxic food additive as a control substance to determine whether you are testable, instead of testing yourself with your left palm over your belly button. For instance, the artificial sweetener aspartame is likely to be harmful to most everyone (since it is comprised of chemicals), so it can be used for this purpose.

If the aspartame causes you to fall back on your heels when you hold it up to your abdomen or chest with your eyes closed, then it means that you are testable, as falling back is your body's way of indicating that a substance is harmful for you. Nearly everyone should have an allergenic-like or toxic response to aspartame!

> In addition to muscle testing for different substances, you can also ask your body "yes" and "no" questions. It will provide a strong muscle response for the "yes" answers and a weak one for the "no" answers.

When testing a nutritional supplement, food or remedy using the standing test, hold the substance against the center of your body with one hand as you stand with your eyes closed. You can place the thing to be tested anywhere between your belly button and chin.

As you do this, observe whether you lean forwards or backwards or don't move at all. A substance that causes you to fall back on your heels is not beneficial for you. If the substance causes you to lean forward, it probably is beneficial. If the substance doesn't cause you to fall back or lean forward, you are likely able to tolerate it, but it is not necessarily beneficial or essential for you.

When you first start this type of testing, you may not notice any obvious movement in your standing position. This is because sometimes the changes are subtle and muscle testing often requires a lot of practice before you are able to consistently discern the slight changes in your body's responses to things.

Also, your mental and emotional biases to the things that you are testing can affect the outcome of the testing. For this reason, it's better to have a friend, family member, or ideally, a health care practitioner, test you while you close your eyes, so that you will not know what they are testing on you.

The standing test is just one of many types of muscle tests that can be used to determine whether you are testable, as well as for testing substances themselves.

The Bi-Digital O-Ring Test (BDORT) is another useful self-test, especially if you want to discreetly or quickly test something such as a food in the supermarket. This test is also best done with a partner, but you can sometimes get fairly accurate results by self-testing if you are able to remove any mental biases that you have about the test results or outcome.

> **Muscle testing takes practice in order to see consistently accurate results. If you see practitioners who use muscle testing in their practice, make sure that they are competent and experienced in their use of it.**

For this test, make an 'O' with either your left or right forefinger and thumb, holding your forefinger and thumb firmly together. At the same time, hold the substance that you want to test against your abdomen. Then, ask your tester to try to pull your finger and thumb apart using his or her forefinger.

If the tester has difficulty doing this because there is strong resistance between your finger and thumb, then it means that the substance that you are testing is likely to be beneficial for you, since your muscle response is strong.

If the substance is harmful, then your finger and thumb will easily come apart when your tester tries to pull them apart. If you are self-testing, you will need to find a way to hold the food, supplement or other object that you are testing against your body, since you'll need to have both of your hands free to do the test.

Whenever you do muscle tests that require you to push or press on a muscle, such as the O-ring test, don't use excessive force upon the muscles that you are using for the testing. Be firm and consistent, but not overly strong.

There is another test that you can do on your own, without the aid of a partner. For this one, move your tongue from side to side in your mouth as fast as you can. Then, to make sure that you are testable, hold some aspartame or other allergenic or toxic control substance against the core of your body or abdomen, to see if your tongue slows down.

If it does, then it means that your body didn't like the aspartame and that you are testable, since your body should produce an allergic/toxic response to aspartame. Slowed tongue movement indicates that your body does not need or like something. If the pace of your tongue remains the same or increases, then it means that whatever you are testing is either neutral or beneficial for your body.

If you have a partner to help you test, there is another test that you can do from home. For this one, lie down on a table or bed and make sure that your body isn't lying over a geopathic field.

Ask your partner to stand at the foot of the table or bed and put his or her thumbs under the bony prominences of your ankles (the place where the ankles nearly touch each other when you are lying down with your feet together). Your partner should place his or her thumbs side-by-side over those bony prominences to determine which of the thumbs is higher, and therefore, closer to your head than the other (and how much closer).

The position of your partner's thumbs will give them an idea about which of your legs is longer. If your body isn't stressed by an allergen, and you aren't lying on a geopathic field, then your legs should be the same length. If one of your legs is normally longer than the other, due to a hip or back misalignment, then your partner will simply want to look for any change in your leg length after you place the substance to be tested on your body.

Usually, when you place something harmful or allergenic on top of your body, one of your legs will appear to become even shorter in relation to the other leg. If you remove the allergen or toxin and your legs become more equal in length, then you know that the allergen or toxin was causing your body to respond negatively.

In addition to muscle testing for different substances, you can also ask your body "yes" and "no" questions, and it will provide a strong muscle response for the "yes" answers, and a weak one for the "no" answers. This test can be done either standing or sitting. The autonomic nervous system, which energetically controls all unconscious functions of your body, knows what is good for your body and what is not.

So, for instance, you can ask your body such questions as, "Do I have a Vitamin C deficiency? Will this vitamin supplement benefit me? Am I allergic to sardines? Can I eat strawberries?" If you test your body using statements rather than physical substances, it's a good idea to verify the answers to those questions by also asking an opposite question, or making an opposite statement, to see if you get an opposite response, as you should if you are testing correctly.

For instance, if you want to test yourself to see if you have an allergy to raisins, you might first say, "I don't have an allergy to raisins." And then say, "I do have an allergy to raisins." If you get the exact opposite response, then you know that your energy isn't blocked and that you are probably testing yourself properly. If you have never asked your body yes and no questions before, then your muscle test results are more likely to be inaccurate in the beginning, until you gain more experience testing.

Some people believe that muscle testing is based upon psychic or spiritual energy, but nothing could be further from the truth. Muscle testing is based upon the physiological energy of the body. It is measurable, electromagnetic energy that comes from the body itself and not an outside entity.

Many integrative and holistic healthcare practitioners are skilled in different forms of muscle testing, such as Autonomic Response Testing (ART) and Contact Reflex Analysis (CRA). These are valid testing techniques but they only work reliably if the practitioner is skilled in their use. ART practitioners can be found either by doing an Internet search using the term "Autonomic Response Testing," along with your city and state, or by contacting The Klinghardt Academy: *KlinghardtAcademy.com.* CRA practitioners can be found by doing an Internet search by using the term "Contact Reflex Analysis."

Muscle testing takes practice in order to see consistently accurate results, so if you see a practitioner who uses muscle testing in their practice, make sure that they are competent and experienced in their use of it. In the meantime, we encourage you to try some of the do-it-yourself techniques at home!

CHAPTER ELEVEN

Electrodermal Screening (EDS)

Electrodermal screening (EDS) is another valuable bioenergetic testing tool that can help you to identify what your body needs. Many practitioners of integrative and alternative medicine use EDS as an aid to help diagnose and treat their patients.

> One advantage of the ZYTO over traditional methods of diagnosis is that it has programs to detect problems in your body that no lab test has yet been designed for.

EDS measures the electrical resistance on your skin's surface and, based on this resistance, detects energy imbalances in your body. These imbalances provide insights into problems that you might have in your organs, systems and tissues, as well as information about nutritional imbalances, toxins or infections.

Electrodermal testing devices, like muscle testing, come in many forms, and measure the body's energy through a variety of means. Electrodermal screening is also known by other names in the integrative medical community, such as limbic stress assessment (LSA), meridian energy analysis (MEA), Bioelectric Functions Diagnosis (BFD), bio-resonance therapy (BRT), computerized electrodermal screening (CEDS), and computerized electrodermal stress analysis (CEDSA).

By measuring the variability in the time interval between your heartbeats, which are controlled by the autonomic nervous system, practitioners of Heart Rate Variability (HRV) can obtain a broad range of information about your health. HRV is a useful tool that can measure and detect stress and problems in your body when other parameters, such as your blood pressure, are normal.

One of the first devices to be developed in Europe was called the Vega. The Prognose, Mora, Listen, Biomeridian, Computron and Interro (for interrogation) are some others. The Interro was developed in the US. These are all classified as point testing devices, which basically means that the person to be tested holds a probe or electrode of the device in one hand, while the tester presses another probe against an acupuncture point (usually on the hand or foot) on the body of the person being tested. To get accurate results with these devices, the practitioner must be very skilled and objective in their use. These are the most common types of electrodermal testing devices.

Another type of device, the galvanic skin device, relies less upon the skill of the technician for accuracy than most other types of electrodermal testing devices, and as such, is more universally effective and reliable in its results. Just like conventional blood, urine and other types of tests, no device provides 100 percent accuracy, but galvanic skin devices generally have a higher level of reliability than any type of point testing device.

All tissues of the body, including the skin, conduct electricity. Electrical energy conductance through the skin is constantly changing and can be measured and charted. The skin's electrical conductivity fluctuates based upon what is going on in the body, and this fluctuation is referred to as the "galvanic skin response."

A lie detector is an example of a galvanic skin response device. When a person is interrogated with questions that create a stress response in their body, the autonomic nerve response on their skin changes and they perspire more, which then increases the electrical conductivity through their skin.

The body's physiological response to stress informs the interrogator that the person being tested is being stressed by what is said, and therefore, possibly lying. In a similar manner, the galvanic skin response devices that are often used in integrative medicine "ask questions"—not with words, but by broadcasting informational signals from the computer's memory into the testing environment.

The ZYTO system is one example of a computerized, semi-automated electrodermal screening device that doctors and other practitioners in the US commonly use. We highly recommend this device, which can help you to discover the source of any problems in your body. It is great because a nurse, technician, or even the office receptionist can scan you with the device and get the same results that a doctor would, because it doesn't require the tester to have a special set of skills in order to get accurate results. The ZYTO can help you to discover a multitude of energetic imbalances and health conditions in your body that lab tests might otherwise miss.

Another advantage of the ZYTO over traditional methods of diagnosis is that it has programs to detect problems in your body that no lab test has yet been designed for.

For instance, conventional labs can only test for a few species of *Borrelia*, one of the most common organisms found in chronic Lyme disease, the fastest-growing infectious disease in the United States. A ZYTO, however, can detect the energetic pattern of more than two dozen species of *Borrelia*. These energetic patterns can indicate whether a particular species of the organism is present in your body, whereas most conventional labs can only detect a few species, and then only some of the time!

Galvanic skin devices can also measure imbalances, deficiencies and excesses in your body. For instance, the ZYTO will reveal if you have an organ that is stressed, or if your hormones are imbalanced, and if so, which ones. It can tell you whether you likely have infections in your body, or emotional stressors, as well as many other things.

The technology is so specific that, for instance, it can tell you which of your teeth are infected with bacteria. It can also identify the specific supplements, drugs and other treatments that are likely to be helpful for healing your body, based on your unique biochemistry. It matches your body chemistry, problems and conditions to the proper remedies.

We highly recommend electrodermal screening and muscle testing as adjunct testing tools to help you to heal from your current health condition, or to simply maintain or improve your well-being. When used along with conventional blood, urine and other types of lab tests, EDS can provide profound insights into the health of your body. EDS, among several others, represents one of the most important, effective and widely used testing methods in bioenergetic medicine.

To find a practitioner in your area that does this type of testing, we recommend doing an Internet search using terms such as "Electrodermal screening" (and then input your city and state) or "ZYTO testing" (city and state).

CHAPTER TWELVE

Heart Rate Variability (HRV) Testing

Heart Rate Variability (HRV) testing is another fantastic evaluative bioenergetic tool that we highly recommend if you want to learn more about your current state of wellness and the cause of any symptoms that you may have. Contrary to how it may sound, HRV testing isn't necessarily used just to evaluate the condition of your heart, but rather, your entire body.

> Like heart rate variability testing (HRV), contact regulation thermography can provide a lot of information about your body by measuring just one parameter of your body—its temperature response to a cold stimulus!

By measuring the variability in the time interval between your heartbeats, which are controlled by the autonomic nervous system, practitioners of HRV can obtain a broad range of information about your health. HRV is a useful tool that can measure and detect stress and problems in your body when other parameters, such as your blood pressure, are normal. With HRV testing, practitioners can discern problems in your body that other tests might miss.

Scientific evidence has shown that people that have high heart rate variability, or great variation in the time interval between their heartbeats tend to be in better health. People who have decreased variability tend to have more health problems, stress and fatigue.

The Heart Quest (HQ) is one particularly useful type of heart rate variability technology that goes beyond simply measuring heart rate variability. According to one of the developers of HQ, Dr. Michael Kessler, in his introductory video on Heart Quest: hrvhq.com, HQ doesn't just measure the function of your autonomic nervous system (or the "automatic" nervous system), as most heart rate variability devices do, but also measures all of your body's regulatory systems, including such things as the neurotransmitters and hormones, and the function and balance of the organs and meridians.

With Heart Quest, practitioners can evaluate whether your health is getting better or worse, and also judge how effective different therapies are for you. Heart Quest can even estimate your physiological age with a fair amount of accuracy. Many of us who are middle-aged or older would prefer to be younger physiologically than we are chronologically, and fortunately we can be, by doing the right things for our health. We can then determine how effective we are at achieving this by following up with this objective test.

If you believe yourself to be healthy, HRV testing is a valuable tool that you can use to verify that you are as healthy as you think. If you are sick, it can help you to determine the source of your illness, and evaluate treatments that would be effective for your recovery.

If the HRV test reveals that you have a diseased organ or other problem in your body, we suggest that you follow up with ZYTO electrodermal testing and/or muscle testing, which can help you to determine the treatments that you would need for that problem. Then, once you have used that treatment for a specified amount of time, we recommend doing another HRV test to see whether or not the treatment benefited you.

One advantage of the HRV over some other types of testing is that it will often reveal positive changes in your body, before those changes can be detected on these other tests or before you notice changes in your symptoms. It can help to confirm the source of your symptoms, along with the ZYTO and other testing devices.

CHAPTER THIRTEEN

Contact Regulation Thermography (CRT) and Chinese Pulse Testing

Contact regulation thermography (CRT) is another great evaluative tool in bioenergetic medicine that can give you information about all of your organ systems. Among the things that CRT reveals include: your body's metabolic activity, levels of inflammation, tissue/organ degeneration, dental stress, lymphatic health, breast or prostate anomalies, heavy metal toxicity and intestinal

> **One of the advantages of CRT (Contact Regulation Thermograpy) over some other types of testing is that it can reveal areas of your body where disease is starting to develop, even life-threatening diseases like cancer, long before the disease shows up on other conventional tests.**

dysfunction. But, like heart rate variability testing, contact regulation thermography can provide a lot of information about your body by measuring just one parameter of your body—its temperature response to a cold stimulus!

In CRT, a computerized screen displays an image of twenty-five of your organs, tissues and systems. For the testing, you stand in a cool room in your underclothes, while a CRT technician applies a sensitive temperature probe to different areas of your body.

> We don't recommend that you entirely substitute conventional tests with energetic tests; there is a time and place for conventional tests. But we believe that energetic tests can often provide a broader overall picture of what is going on in your body, and at a fraction of the cost, in less time, and with less hassle than conventional medical testing.

With the probe, the technician measures your skin temperature at up to 119 locations (each of which corresponds to a particular organ system) first immediately after you take your clothes off and then again after you are exposed to the cool room for a few minutes. This is done to monitor changes in your circulation and autonomic nervous system.

The difference in your body's temperature, both before and after the cold stimulus test, reveals how well your organs and tissues are functioning, and how well your body handles stress. For instance, if you have a problem in a particular organ or tissue, the skin temperature in that area will not fluctuate much when you are exposed to cold.

In a healthy person, a cold stimulus will cause blood vessels to constrict, and blood to be shunted away from the skin and associated organs, so that the skin area becomes cold. In someone who has diseased organs and tissues, this process doesn't happen as effectively.

One of the advantages of CRT over some other types of testing is that it can reveal areas of your body where disease is starting to develop, even life-threatening diseases like cancer, long before the disease shows up on other conventional tests. As such, CRT can be a useful tool for disease prevention or for catching disease in the early stages.

Because of this, we highly recommend CRT testing as part of a comprehensive wellness or disease prevention protocol. It is an easy, painless way to get a regular check-up without having to do a lot of blood, urine or other conventional tests. Even if you feel perfectly well, CRT can reveal potential weak spots in your body that might eventually cause you trouble, so that you can take extra steps to keep that part of you well.

Ideally, we recommend doing Contact Regulation Thermography on a yearly basis. If the tester finds a significant abnormality on your annual CRT, you might consider doing a follow-up CRT after undergoing therapy or treatment for that condition. You can find practitioners that use CRT by visiting: *alfathermo. com* or *eidam.com.*

Chinese Pulse Testing

Chinese pulse testing is another wonderful diagnostic tool in bioenergetic medicine. For this, a doctor trained in Traditional Chinese Medicine checks for any health problems in your body by taking your pulses. Isn't it interesting how one physiological parameter, such as body temperature, heart rate variability or the pulse, can reveal so much about the body? We think so!

Chinese or oriental medical doctors have used pulse testing as a diagnostic tool for over 2000 years. Pulse taking provides energetic information about your body that correlates with specific anatomical and biochemical information. This information helps doctors to identify disease and areas of weakness in your body.

When an oriental medical doctor takes your pulse, they place their right index, middle and ring fingers on the radial artery of your left wrist, and the left index, middle and ring fingers on your right radial artery.

> If your current wellness strategies aren't working or doing enough to bring you to optimum health, we invite you to try out some healing tools in bioenergetic medicine.

With these six fingers, they feel the pulse characteristics of your body on both wrists simultaneously, as they press both lightly and firmly on each wrist. Each finger that is used in the testing process is used to test two different organ systems in your body. All twelve of your body's primary organ systems can be assessed in this way.

Doctors that do pulse testing study the characteristics of the pulse, which can be slow, feathery, forceful, stressed—or any number of things. With pulse testing, experienced doctors can tell you 120 different things about your body just by holding your radial (wrist) pulses for two to three minutes.

If you are intuitive, you can learn to self-test your pulses. For most of us, however, it's just important to know that if our conventional, western-minded medical doctors can't figure out what's wrong with us, then it may be beneficial for us to visit a traditional Chinese medical doctor, who can, by pulse testing, often identify a problem in our bodies that other doctors have missed.

SUMMARY OF BIOENERGETIC TESTING

Most of us are accustomed to relying upon conventional medical tests such as blood, urine, stool or saliva tests, as well as various types of X-ray procedures, to diagnose disease and determine our overall state of wellness. These tests, while important, cannot measure everything that is going on in our bodies, and fall far short of providing the "big picture" about what is happening inside of us.

You can find practitioners that use CRT by visiting: *alfathermo.com* or *eidam.com*.

We can fill in the gaps with energetic testing devices and techniques, which can detect a multitude of problems in the body, all within a single testing session, and with immediate results.

We don't recommend that you substitute conventional tests entirely with energetic tests; there is a time and place for conventional tests. But we believe that energetic tests can often provide a broader overall picture of what's going on in your body, at a fraction of the cost, in less time, and with less hassle than conventional medical testing.

They are, therefore, essential tools for helping you to stay healthy and prevent disease, as well as for helping you to heal from disease. We recommend finding a healthcare practitioner that utilizes one or two of the tools that we have described in this part of the book to assess your current state of health.

To do this, pick one, two or more of the testing modalities that we mentioned in this section—depending on your energy, time and finances—and do an Internet search on those testing modalities. When you do this, be sure to input your city and state in the search box as well. This will usually bring up a list of practitioners in your state that use these tools, or at least their websites.

Next, ask the nutritionist or other employee at your local health food store for advice about the practitioners that you found in your Internet search. Chances are they have heard about them and know about the kinds of services they can provide, as well as their reputations. Then make an appointment with one of the practitioners based on the information that you have gathered.

You'll likely be amazed at what you learn from these evaluations, and how much better equipped you will be to heal from whatever ails you, or to maintain your current state of wellness.

If you happen to visit a practitioner that wants to recommend a treatment that is unfamiliar to you, you may want to first gather as much information as you can about that recommended treatment(s) before starting it. Much of what is written on the Internet about treatments is inaccurate; we therefore suggest doing research using a variety of resources.

CHAPTER FOURTEEN

Suzy's Story

Suzy had tried it all—physical therapy, chiropractic adjustments, Rolfing, Pilates, yoga and ten different pain medications. She had seen osteopathic, chiropractic and medical doctors, along with an assortment of therapists and teachers, and still, her neck and back pain from the car accident was unrelenting.

She had read on the Internet about pulsed electromagnetic field (PEMF) therapy for pain, but didn't know if it would be a worthwhile investment. After all, she had already spent thousands of dollars, and seen every practitioner under the sun. Still, she had read that PEMF therapy could actually help bones and tissues to heal, while reducing inflammation.

Some of the other treatments that she had done seemed to only temporarily relieve her symptoms, rather than heal her body. How would she even find a practitioner? PEMF therapy seemed expensive, but if it worked, it would cost a lot less than what she had already spent for the multitude of chiropractic, physician and pain treatments that she had already done.

If you've ever suffered from pain, you might be able to relate to Suzy's story of "trying it all," spending thousands of dollars, and experiencing only mild to moderate relief of your symptoms—if any!

Fortunately, bioenergetic medicine offers lots of safe and effective strategies, gadgets and remedies for pain relief, such as PEMF therapy, as well as for a multitude of other health conditions. If your current wellness strategies aren't working or doing enough to bring you to optimum health, we invite you to try out some healing tools in bioenergetic medicine.

In the following chapters, we describe those that we have found to be most effective for relieving five of today's most common conditions—fatigue, pain, insomnia, depression and anxiety.

We chose the five above-mentioned conditions for this book because who hasn't suffered from fatigue, pain, insomnia, depression or anxiety at some point during their lifetime? We believe that these are among the most common health conditions that most of us battle today, either occasionally or daily.

However, the tools that we describe in the following chapters can also be used to treat a multitude of other conditions. So if you have another symptom or problem that is not mentioned here, we recommend doing further research on your own to see how these tools might also help you with your particular issue.

The underlying cause of symptoms varies from person to person. For instance, if you suffer from fatigue, it may be due to infections, environmental toxins, heart disease, stress or other factors. For this reason, the benefit that you will get from each of the bioenergetic tools that we describe in this book will depend somewhat upon the underlying cause of your symptoms, as well as your unique biochemistry and physiology.

That said, these treatment tools are useful for alleviating a variety of symptoms, regardless of their cause. After reading this part of the book, we recommend discussing some of these tools with a doctor, preferably a naturopath or integrative healthcare practitioner—and then trying some of them out.

You may find that they will indirectly resolve your underlying illness, lessen your symptoms, or simply improve your feelings of well-being. Because when your energy is balanced, your biochemistry, including that of all your organs and systems, will also come back into alignment. And when your energy is aligned and your chemistry balanced, you will feel great, regardless of the initial cause of your symptoms!

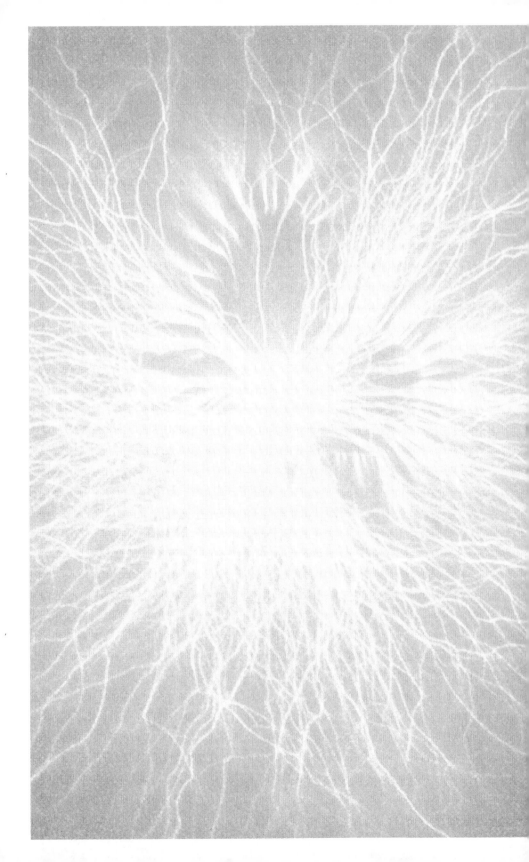

BioEnergetic Treatments
for Fatigue

In the following chapters, we describe several of our favorite and most effective tools for restoring and balancing your energy. We include therapies and remedies that are suitable for people on a budget (but which require a bit more effort and time), as well as those that are suitable for people who have the money, but not the time or inclination to learn new tools or techniques.

Like the diagnostic tools that are described in the first part of this book, these treatment tools include manual, or hands-on therapies, as well as energetic devices, and supplemental remedies.

CHAPTER FIFTEEN

The King Method (TKM®)

Many of us are sluggish, tired or downright exhausted on a daily basis, due to the poor quality of our diets, environmental toxins, infectious disease, emotional stress and a hectic lifestyle, among other things. These stressors can sap our stamina and energy and cause us to feel less than our best.

> The King Method (TKM®) is simply a means to help the body function as God created it to function and heal itself. It is about God's creation and design working properly.

Whether you are moderately sluggish, or exhausted on a daily basis, bioenergetic medicine can be extraordinarily useful for increasing your energy, vitality and stamina. Even if you don't feel that tired, you might appreciate having a bit more energy to accomplish your daily tasks.

The King Method(TKM®) is a hands-on healing technique that is based on the idea that the bio-electromagnetic system of the physical body governs its well-being, and that when this system works well, the body functions properly.

Glenn King, PhD, CDN, CN, and Director of the King Institute, Inc., developed TKM after learning about the physics of the body's bio-electromagnetic system and how it affects human health. TKM is the product of Dr. King's discoveries, spiritual revelations from God, and the studies of others.

The Median Sequence, as well as the other TKM sequences, balances the autonomic nervous system, and with that your body's energy. This, in turn, alleviates fatigue and helps you to relax.

The cultural roots of TKM can be traced to the Orient and perhaps even ancient Greece, although Dr. King credits God with ultimately teaching him how to develop the technique, since his revelations about TKM have resulted from extensive prayer, along with his studies and research.

According to The King Institute website: "The King Institute Method® (TKM®) is an extraordinary hands-on approach to health disorders. This method has been shown to have a profound effect on the bio-electromagnetic systems of the body, which affect all bio-systems. The initial understanding of TKM® has been effectively utilized to treat people for years for common to complex disorders."

According to Dr. King, TKM is not a renaming of any other kind of hands-on therapy, and is a unique method to naturally heal the body. Unlike some other types of hands-on therapy, it does not draw upon outside energies, only your body's innate electromagnetic energy.

> The many sequences involved in TKM take a bit of practice and time to learn, but the basic Median Sequence almost anyone can do, and this one technique alone can go a long way toward increasing your energy.

Also, TKM energy pathways are different from the meridian energy pathways commonly described in bioenergetic medicine. According to Dr. King, there are different levels or densities of energy in the human body, which precede one another. They are also interdependent, connecting with one another. Whereas TKM energy pathways go deeper, meridian energy is a more superficial level of energy circulation in the body.

The King Institute boasts many healing testimonials on its website which demonstrate the effectiveness of TKM for treating a variety of acute and chronic conditions, including low energy. Thousands of people, including many with medically incurable diseases or genetic disorders, have been healed by this unique hands-on therapy, although Dr. King doesn't claim to be a healer and says that TKM® is not a healing method.

Rather, says Dr. King,

"… (TKM®) is simply a means to help the body function as God created it to function and heal itself. It is about God's creation and design working properly. When it doesn't work, then God has provided the knowledge to repair it. The body already has the innate capacity to heal itself, and TKM® is simply a method that encourages the body to do that."

TKM increases your energy by balancing the different energy pathways of your body, and by removing energetic blockages that lead to disease.

This is one of our favorite strategies for increasing energy, vitality and stamina because the techniques are simple, once you learn them, and don't cost you anything to do—just a bit of your time.

While Dr. King has developed TKM techniques for many different disorders, one of the most basic and powerful techniques, called the Median Sequence, is excellent for alleviating fatigue and increasing energy, no matter the cause! You can learn it in just 15 to 30 minutes. Step-by-step instructions for how to do it are outlined below.

How to Do The Median Sequence (A Self-Help Sequence)

Sit, or preferably lie, in a comfortable position. To get the best results, remove all metallic objects from your body and clothing, including underwire bras, watches, belts and jewelry. It's best to wear 100 percent cotton clothing that has all of its synthetic labels removed, and to position pillows beneath your arms, so that your muscles can completely relax as you apply each step of the procedure.

For this sequence, you will be placing the pads of your first three fingers (index, middle, and ring), palm side down, on different points (areas) of your body. Or, if you wish, you may use all of your finger pads.

The Median Sequence
(Sequence for Self-Help)

Preparation: Sit, or preferably lie, in a comfortable position. For best results remove all metallic objects from the body and from clothing. 100% cotton clothing is best suited. It is suggested to position pillows beneath arms as needed in order to completely relax while applying each step of the procedure.

Length of time: Hold each step (location) a minimum of four to five minutes, or up to twenty minutes if needed.

Application: Use the pads (palm side down) of your first three fingers (index, middle, and ring) to apply contact with any location. Or, you may use all fingers (pads) if you wish.

Always hold two locations simultaneously when applying a sequence, one with each hand.

Important: Pressure is not necessary to achieve results. In fact, it may inhibit the process. Contact is all that is needed to stimulate energy circulation.

When to apply: We suggest first thing in the morning before rising from bed and the last of the day when lying in bed. This can be accomplished at other times, however these are the most productive times and are complementary to most schedules. The entire sequence usually takes approximately thirty to forty minutes for proper results. Refer to Figure 11.

Figure 11

Sequence Steps:

Procedure For the Hands	(to)	Positions On the Body		
			1st	RIGHT LEFT
			2nd	LEFT
Step 1 Place right hand's fingers	to	Top center of Head		
and Place left hand's fingers	to	Center of the Forehead *(above and between eyebrows)*	3rd	LEFT
Step 2 Place left hand's fingers	to	Tip of the Nose *(very light touch)*	4th	LEFT
Step 3 Place left hand's fingers	to	Center of Collarbone *(center on interclavicular notch)*	5th	LEFT
Step 4 Place left hand's fingers	to	Center of the Chest *(on sternum at center of gladiolus)*		
Step 5 Place left hand's fingers	to	Bottom of Sternum *(tip of sternum, or xiphoid appendix)*	6th	LEFT
Step 6 Place left hand's fingers	to	Umbilicus *(Navel)*	7th	LEFT
Step 7 Place left hand's fingers	to	Center of Pubic Bone *(above and against the top center of pubic bone)*		
Step 8 Place right hand's fingers	to	Coccyx *(tip of tail bone)*	8th	RIGHT

The procedure helps the autonomic nervous system and all organs and their bioelectromagnetic energy. It helps calm the mind, relieve stress, relax the body, and rejuvenate and balance the body's bioelectromagnetic energy conductivity. It is an excellent preventative medicine practice and assists the body in correcting acute and chronic health disorders. This procedure has produced powerful results for the overall body through this simple application. Therefore, this procedure is a high priority for a healthy life or health recovery.

This sequence also opens, strengthens, and balances the main bioelectromagnetic energy circulation which allows TKM® procedures applied afterwards to be much more effective to help physical, mental, and emotional health needs.

Start by placing the pads of your right fingers on the top of your head in your midline, while simultaneously and sequentially placing the pads of your left fingers on each of the following points on the front midline of your body, as indicated by the diagram on the previous page.

Leave your fingers on each of these points for 4 to 5 minutes (although you can obtain better results by leaving them there for up to 20 minutes per point), while keeping your right fingers on the top of your head. Four to five minutes after you get to the last point on the front of your body (the pubic bone), remove your right fingers from the top of your head and place them on your tailbone, while keeping your left fingers on the pubic bone (the last location).

As you do this, it is not necessary that you apply pressure to your skin with your fingers; in fact, this can inhibit the healing process. Contacting your body (even through a single layer of clothing) is all that is needed to stimulate energy circulation.

To obtain the maximum benefit from TKM, we suggest doing the Median Sequence first thing in the morning before you arise, and at the end of the day, when you are lying in bed. You can do it at other times of the day as well, but morning and night are usually the most convenient and doing it at bedtime can help you to fall asleep more easily.

According to the King Institute website (*kinginstitute.org*), the Median Sequence, as well as the other TKM sequences, balance the autonomic nervous system, and with that, your body's energy. This, in turn, alleviates fatigue and helps you to relax. Among other benefits, it also calms your mind, relieves stress, and relaxes and rejuvenates you.

While we recommend the Median Sequence for increasing energy, in reality, TKM can do much more for you besides this. Here we only describe the most basic (although one of the most powerful!) sequences for increasing your energy. There are others as well.

Dr. King has developed other TKM sequences that can help heal the body of many kinds of serious chronic and degenerative conditions. Testimonials of healing from these conditions can be found on the TKM website:

kinginstitute.org/services/testimonials.html

The King Institute also offers training courses for people that are interested in becoming TKM practitioners, or who simply want to learn the techniques to use on themselves or their family and friends. The many sequences involved in TKM take a bit of practice and time to learn, but the basic Median Sequence almost anyone can do, and this one technique alone can go a long way toward increasing your energy (by balancing it) and even improving other symptoms of disease that you might have.

Many of the TKM techniques are best done with a partner, and you can sometimes get faster results this way, since there are four hands involved in the techniques, instead of two.

I have recommended and used TKM extensively on my patients. In TKM, each hand acts like a jumper cable and moves stagnant energy from "upstream," in an energy pathway where it's not supposed to be, to downstream, where it is needed. The position of your hands causes your body to redistribute energy to where it's most needed.

Also, I have found that when you do the TKM sequences, it's a good idea to touch the roof of your mouth with your tongue, as this helps to ensure an effective flow of energy throughout your body. If you have chronic fatigue, and you do this Median Sequence twice daily, once at night and once again during the day, over time you will notice your energy reserves increasing.

In the early 1990s, I had several hundred patients in my practice that were completely disabled from severe chronic fatigue. Statistics have shown that more than 70 percent of people with chronic fatigue will never become well enough to return to work. I found, however, that 80 percent of my chronic fatigue patients that consistently did TKM, drank sufficient amounts of pure water, ate mostly raw, whole foods, and detoxified their bodies, recovered their health and returned to work after just a few months.   —Dr. Lee Cowden

CHAPTER SIXTEEN

Pulsed Electromagnetic Field Therapy (PEMF)

Pulsed Electromagnetic Field (PEMF) therapy is another great therapy that we recommend for increasing your energy and vitality, and which is becoming increasingly popular in the United States. PEMF therapy usually involves treating your body with a device that uses a pulsating electromagnetic field to create currents that have a beneficial effect upon your energy field. There are many types of PEMF devices, but for the purposes of this book we will only be describing a few that we have found to be useful for promoting energy and well-being.

> **Studies have proven that the entire body responds positively when exposed to the proper frequency and intensity of pulsed electromagnetic fields. This includes the bone marrow, blood, muscle, ligaments, bone, cartilage and organs.**

Studies have proven that the entire body responds positively when exposed to the proper frequency and intensity of pulsed electromagnetic fields. This includes the bone marrow, blood, muscle, ligaments, bone, cartilage and organs. When you use the proper energetic field frequency and intensity, PEMF therapy can improve or even resolve serious health conditions and diseases.

Usually the benefits of PEMF therapy manifest immediately. In addition to having more energy, people often report improved cognition, emotional well-being and sleep, as well as less pain after just a session or two of treatment.

PEMF therapy can increase your energy and eliminate fatigue by reducing inflammation; opening up your circulation, increasing your blood and tissue oxygenation and nutrient uptake; improving cellular detoxification (or garbage removal from your cells) and regeneration; and enhancing your quality of rest.

Also, PEMF therapy increases energy by improving the transmembrane electrical potential of your cells so that they function properly again. A highly negative transmembrane electrical potential correlates with good energy, healthy cellular function, and the ability of the cells to uptake nutrients and remove waste.

The tiny structures inside of your cell, which are called organelles, also have a transmembrane electrical potential (especially the mitochondrial organelles which produce most of the cell's energy). The cellular organelles function much like the organs of your body; they are to the cells what the organs are to the body.

The mitochondria, golgi bodies and other organelles inside of the cell all have membranes, like the cell itself, and the membranes that enclose them also have a transmembrane electrical potential. So when the cell's transmembrane potential, or that of the organelles is low, then the cell can't provide energy to the body or repair itself. This can lead to a variety of diseases and health problems.

PEMF therapy can help to create energy by regenerating your cells and even heal your body of disease by restoring the transmembrane electrical potential in your cells as well as possibly that of the cell's organelles.

PEMF can, therefore, be a great therapy, even life-saving, if you are profoundly energy depleted. People who are chronically ill or very tired often don't have enough energetic charge in their cells to be able to produce a healing response in their bodies. So for such people, using PEMF can kind of be like taking a car that won't start because the battery is dead, and plugging it into a super-charger for a few minutes.

> The Earth's natural frequency and its beneficial effects upon our bodies have been drowned out by the much higher, more dangerous frequencies of AC power lines, home and office appliances, cell phones, cell phone towers, wireless Internet, radio and TV stations.

Among its other benefits, PEMF therapy can normalize your blood pressure and cholesterol levels, balance your immune system, relax your body and if you have an injury or wound, accelerate bone and soft tissue repair.

One advantage of PEMF therapy over TKM is that it requires less effort than TKM (you usually just lie on a mat or sit next to or on some other type of PEMF device for five to twenty-five minutes), but it can be more expensive than TKM, which may be an important consideration if you are on a tight budget.

Also, you can harm your body if you overdo it and use an incorrect frequency or treat yourself for too long. For that reason, we might recommend TKM if you are very sensitive to electromagnetic fields, or don't have a lot of money to spend, and PEMF if you don't have a lot of time to do treatments, but have a bit more money to spend and someone who can guide you in the use of the devices.

Fortunately, PEMF devices, such as therapeutic mats, have become more affordable in recent years. These can be purchased online for at-home use.

Another advantage of PEMF therapy is that it often lessens the need to do or take other health remedies, like nutritional supplements. This is because this therapy, like TKM, balances your body's energy, causing a multitude of biochemical processes to become more efficient. PEMF can even increase nutrient uptake into the cells (via a process called electroporation).

Therefore, PEMF is also useful for healing your body of a wide variety of health conditions, with an increase in energy and stamina being one of its primary benefits.

PEMF therapy has been around for decades, although it hasn't been used much in conventional medicine, except to treat pain and accelerate wound healing, for which it is also extremely useful. Lately, its use has become more widespread in integrative medicine.

Usually the benefits of PEMF therapy manifest immediately. In addition to having more energy, people often report improved cognition, emotional well-being and sleep, as well as less pain after just a session or two of treatment.

Long-term healing from chronic health conditions can take months to accomplish with PEMF therapy, however. Also, if you have a high burden of environmental toxins in your body or are seriously ill, PEMF therapy can cause you to initially feel worse for a period of several days to weeks, as it causes your body to mobilize environmental toxins out of your cells. But if you start out slowly with this therapy, doing it for just a few minutes per day, you may be able to avoid this detoxification response and the symptoms that come along with that.

Over the long term, if you use the right frequencies for an adequate amount of time, PEMF therapy can eliminate fatigue and be a powerful adjunct (supportive therapy) for healing from a variety of chronic and degenerative diseases, including chronic fatigue syndrome, Lyme disease, fibromyalgia, arthritis, and cancer.

Types of PEMF Devices

PEMF devices come in many different forms and types, and range from mats, probes and pads, to plastic rings and cylinders that you either lie on or place somewhere on or near to your body. These devices generate magnetic fields that are pulsed using different waveforms at a variety of frequencies and intensities. Most of these products are relatively easy to use.

Some of the more effective PEMF devices tend to use earth frequencies known as Tesla-Shumann resonance (around eight Hertz) and their harmonics (multiples of the eight Hz frequency). Eight Hertz (eight cycles per second) is the optimal frequency of a contemplative human brain. The natural frequency of the earth is 7.83 Hz—close to eight Hz.

Unfortunately, the Earth's natural frequency and its beneficial effects upon our bodies has been drowned out by the much higher, more dangerous frequencies of AC power lines, home and office appliances, cell phones, cell phone towers, wireless Internet, radio and TV stations, as well as other sources, making it much harder for our bodies to function properly.

A Rife machine is a PEMF device that delivers electromagnetic frequencies to your body, which are specific for eliminating disease-causing microbes or strengthening weakened organs. In doing this, it can also increase your energy.

One type of useful PEMF device that we recommend for at-home use is a PEMF mat, which you can buy online from a variety of retailers. PEMF mats contain coils of wire that are energized by controller units that pulse electromagnetic fields through your body. You can often rent one of these mats for a week or month before you decide to buy one. They are useful for balancing your energy and alleviating fatigue. Below we recommend a few types of mats that have been proven, anecdotally and/or in research studies, to be relatively safe and effective.

These mats include the Mediconsult iMRS/MRS2000, Magnafield and BEMER. The BEMER might have the most research studies to back its effectiveness and safety, and is a decent choice for that reason. These studies can be found on the *PubMed.org* medical research database, as well as on the BEMER website: *BemerAmerica.com/BemerGroup/why-bemer/scientifically-proven/*

Another good choice is the Magnafield, which has been used in Australia for about 20 years and is manufactured by Magnacare in the United Kingdom. For more information on the Magnafield, visit: *MagnaCareUK.com.*

A third option is the iMRS, which has been used in Europe for more than twenty years and currently has millions of users worldwide. It has been proven anecdotally to be safe for many people, when it's used correctly. For more information on the iMRS, see: *imrs.com.*

While these mats can provide fantastic health benefits to the body, not everyone responds positively to them, especially people that have a chronic illness and/or electromagnetic sensitivities. For this reason, if you choose to do this type of therapy, we recommend starting out very slowly and using the mat for no more than a few minutes daily, especially if you are EMF-sensitive or have a chronic health condition. If you purchase your own device, make sure that it's one that has research studies and numerous anecdotal reports of its success verifying its safety and efficacy—such as the BEMER.

Also, it's best to work with someone who can guide you in your treatment sessions, because there are no established treatment regimens for PEMF therapy, and not everyone benefits from the same frequencies, duration and type of treatment.

Dr. Cowden has discovered 38 specific frequencies that are useful for supporting the organs, which you can program into almost any Rife device that has a frequency range of 0 to 100,000 Hz (organ support frequencies are usually between 20,000 to 100,000 Hz).

Most devices that are sold for at-home use cost anywhere from $2000-$4500, with the average cost for a good device costing between $3000 and $4000.

When you do PEMF therapy for energy, it's usually not necessary to use the device for as long a period of time as you would to treat other conditions, such as healing a bone or wound. Using a lower intensity field for just a few minutes per day may be sufficient, although it's difficult to provide specific guidelines here, as the duration of your treatment and the frequencies that you'll need will depend upon the device that you use and your unique biochemistry and physiology.

For at-home treatments, Dr. Cowden prefers the Magnafield devices (or even the Magnatens battery-operated devices) because these devices, instead of using a square-wave waveform, like most other devices on the market, use a complex, clustered spike waveform, which is much closer to the energy waveform that is produced by the human nervous system.

More powerful devices, such as the PMT-100, which Dr. Cowden also recommends, can bring about more dramatic and faster results for some types of conditions, but these are generally much more expensive, usually costing more than $20,000.

Many practitioners use the PMT-100, so you can pay for individual treatment sessions, which cost much less than purchasing the device. Make sure to work with a practitioner that has a strong track record of success in treating people with the device. Unfortunately, there are no established lists of practitioners that use this kind of therapy, so we recommend asking for a referral directly from the PMT-100 vendors at: *PEMF.us* and *PemfforLife.com*.

RIFE MACHINES

A Rife machine is a PEMF device that delivers electromagnetic frequencies to your body which are specific for eliminating disease-causing microbes or strengthening weakened organs. In doing this, it can also increase your energy.

There are different types of Rife machines, and, like all devices, some are more effective than others. You can treat systemic problems in your body with what are called radiant (plasma-tube) instruments, which transmit electromagnetic frequencies into your body from a distance. (Usually this distance is several feet or several meters from your body.) One benefit of using a radiant Rife device is that you can do a variety of other tasks while you are receiving treatment, since you are not connected to the device during treatment.

Other devices, called contact devices, are useful for treating specific organs or parts of your body. They utilize silver-impregnated electrode pads, metallic probes or plates, which you apply directly to your skin, usually over the troubled area.

Rife therapy might be best known for its usefulness in killing microbes that cause infection, but it is also beneficial for increasing energy. It does this by giving a boost to your organs, especially the hormonal glands and detoxification organs, so that they function better.

Most of us have sluggish or overwhelmed detoxification organs, due to the plethora of environmental toxins to which we are exposed daily and which our livers, gallbladders, kidneys, lymphatic system, lungs and skin must continually eliminate. If you use a Rife machine with the correct organ support frequencies, you can strengthen your organs so that they perform their jobs better. In turn, this causes your body to become more efficient and have fewer toxins to eliminate, which then also increases your energy.

Rife therapy can also improve your adrenal and thyroid function, both of which are intimately involved in energy production.

Dr. Cowden has discovered 38 specific frequencies that are useful for supporting the organs, which you can program into almost any Rife device that has a frequency range of 0 to 100,000 Hz (since organ support frequencies are usually between 20,000 to 100,000 Hz). You can access the list of these frequencies by becoming a Premier Member, Healthcare Practitioner Member or Friend Member of the Academy of Comprehensive Integrative Medicine: *ACIMconnect.com.*

Usually the higher frequency Rife devices are more sophisticated and expensive, so you may need to visit a health-care practitioner that does Rife therapy, rather than purchase a device on your own.

That said, there is one type of device that you might find affordable for at-home use, called the PFG-2Z Pulsed Tech device. This is a contact Rife-like device that costs approximately 2000 dollars, and is the cheapest device that has fully programmable frequencies and waveforms. It also has precise enough frequencies to both support the organs and kill mutated microbes.

This device is a great investment because you can use it for years, over and over again, whenever you feel that your body needs an energy boost, or help detoxifying, or getting over an infection. For more information on this device, visit the Pulsed Technologies website: *PulsedTech.com/pfg2z.html.*

Not all Rife devices can be programmed for specific frequencies (they instead contain pre-programmed frequencies), and many don't have frequencies that run higher than 10,000 Hertz (or sometimes even above 1000 Hertz). Others have other limitations or problems that can restrict their effectiveness; therefore, we recommend purchasing only a device that is well recommended by healthcare professionals, such as the PFG-2Z from Pulsed Tech.

CHAPTER SEVENTEEN

Acupuncture/ Laserpuncture/Acupressure

Acupuncture is another great energy-increasing and energy-balancing healing modality that we highly recommend, if you can afford to see an acupuncture practitioner and go to a clinic on a regular basis, or if you just need a one or two session tune-up.

Acupuncture balances the flow of Qi through your body's meridians, and is useful for treating a variety of conditions, including low energy. It increases your energy by improving the function of all of your vital organs and systems.

It is used in Traditional Chinese medicine (TCM) not only to increase energy, but also to treat a multitude of disease conditions. For the purposes of this book, we will be describing why and how it is useful for eliminating fatigue and increasing energy.

The Chinese healing art of acupuncture dates back at least 2000 years. It was developed out of one of the most important concepts of Chinese medicine, which is that of balancing the body. The theory of yin and yang are derived from the concept of balance. According to this theory, all things in life happen in an alternating rhythm of yin and yang, and it's important to balance both. Yin represents the cool, quiet, sedate, predominantly female aspects of health in men and women. Yang represents the warm, boisterous, predominantly male aspects of health in men and women.

According to Traditional Chinese Medicine (TCM), good health is achieved when there is balance and harmony of all that is yin and yang within the body. When there is balance, there is healthy circulation of the body's life force, called Qi (pronounced "chee") in Chinese medicine.

Qi, which some of us in the West might refer to as the body's electromagnetic field, is said to travel through the body along channels called meridians. Qi flows up and down these pathways, and when the flow of Qi is not normal in all of the pathways, yin and yang become imbalanced, and health problems can result.

Acupuncture balances the flow of Qi through your body's meridians and is useful for treating a variety of conditions, including low energy. It increases your energy by improving the function of all of your vital organs and systems, including your heart, circulation, hormonal glands, kidneys, liver, digestive organs and nervous system.

To do acupuncture, a practitioner inserts very fine needles into your skin, sometimes in combination with electricity or heat, which enhances the effects of the needles. Heat is produced by burning specific herbs at acupuncture points through a process called Moxibustion.

There are more than 365 acupuncture points on the body that are commonly used by Chinese acupuncturists, most of which are thought to have a specific energetic function. Some of these points, when stimulated, move energy toward the interior of the body, while others bring energy toward its surface. Whenever acupuncture is done using needles along with electricity or herbs, or by using a low-level laserpuncture or acupressure device, you can get a nice jumpstart to your energy system.

In recent years, acupuncture has become more widely used in Western medicine, which means that it's relatively easy to find a practitioner in most US towns and cities. If you can do acupuncture at a clinic on a regular basis, it can help to temporarily or permanently resolve your fatigue, depending on the cause.

The only drawback to acupuncture is that you can't do it on your own, and you may need to visit a clinic regularly to maintain its benefits if you have a chronic health condition. However, if you study the principles of acupuncture on your own, or understand how the acupoints on the body work, you can sometimes obtain similar benefits by shining a laser light on these points. When a laser is used to treat acupoints, the technique is called laserpuncture. Red lasers stimulate acupoints and blue lasers sedate acupoints.

Another way that you can obtain some of the benefits of acupuncture on you own is by doing simple acupressure or reflexology techniques on your hands or feet.

Simply use your fingertips to press around on different areas of your hands or feet until you find a tender spot. Tender spots indicate stressed organs somewhere in your body, so when you find a spot that is tender, massage that spot in a clockwise circular fashion for a few seconds up to a few minutes until it is no longer tender. By doing this, you can help to balance the energy flow to the stressed organ that corresponds with the spot on your hands or feet. By releasing stress from your organs, you can indirectly increase your energy.

Over time, acupuncture and acupressure can permanently resolve even serious health conditions by balancing your body's energy. In the short-term, they are powerful treatments for increasing your energy.

CHAPTER EIGHTEEN

Other Ways to Eliminate Fatigue and Increase Your Energy and Vitality

In the following sections, we summarize a few other tools that we recommend for increasing your energy, stamina and vitality. We encourage you to research these on your own, since it is beyond the scope of this book to describe every type of bioenergetic healing modality in great detail.

Energetically imprinted herbs can be powerful but gentle remedies for increasing energy. One that we like, called Adrenal Support, is made by the herbal supplement company NutraMedix (*NutraMedix.com*) and is especially useful if your fatigue is caused by stress.

Energetically Imprinted Herbal Remedies

Energetically imprinted herbs can be powerful but gentle remedies for increasing energy. One that we particularly like, called Adrenal Support, is made by the herbal supplement company NutraMedix (*NutraMedix.com*), and is especially useful if your fatigue is caused by stress—whether emotional, physical or mental. Since the adrenal glands are involved in your body's stress response, supporting them with energetically imprinted herbs and nutrients can dramatically increase your energy.

> No matter the cause of your pain, bioenergetic medicine provides some excellent and safe alternatives to drugs and other therapies. And unlike drugs, it can often help to heal your body and remove the underlying cause of your pain, rather than just temporarily alleviate your symptoms.

Adrenal Support is a proprietary blend of five adaptogenic herbs that support adrenal gland function: schizandra, astragalus, rhododendron, ginseng and rhodiola. This product, as well as others by NutraMedix, are also energetically imprinted with frequencies that support organ function and proper energy flow throughout the body.

In the *Bioenergetic Treatments for Anxiety* section of this book, we explain the concept of homeopathy and energetically imprinted remedies in greater depth, and how they work to promote wellness.

(Disclosure: Dr. Cowden is a paid consultant to NutraMedix; however, he recommends the NutraMedix products because he has had more success in using them on his patients than other remedies. That said, he encourages you to try similar products from other companies as well.)

EARTHING

Earthing involves connecting your body to the Earth's natural energetic frequencies, which you can do either by standing barefoot outside, or by contacting your skin with special conductive devices, such as metallic-lined Earthing sheets that ground you to the earth through the grounding plug in the electrical outlets in your home.

With Earthing, the direct current of the earth (electrons) flows into your body, and quenches free radicals, reduces inflammation and causes the spontaneous release of toxins from your tissues.

In "Earthing" (contacting your body directly with the Earth), the current of the earth (electrons) flows into your body, quenching free radicals, reducing inflammation and causing the spontaneous release of toxins from your tissues.

You can sleep grounded to the earth by using an Earthing sheet on your bed, which is attached by a wire to a plug that fits into the grounding socket of an electrical outlet.

If you choose to use an Earthing sheet, we recommend that you start by lying on the sheet for only 15 minutes the first night and building up incrementally by 15 minutes per night, since aligning your energy with the earth's can cause your cells to spontaneously detoxify. You don't want to mobilize so many toxins from your tissues that you make yourself ill, which is why it's a good idea to start out slowly.

Earthing, like all of the therapies in this book, restores proper energy balance to your body, resulting in more energy, deeper sleep, less inflammation, and other improvements to your overall well-being. For more information on Earthing, and Earthing products, such as Earthing sheets, we encourage you to visit the Earthing website: *EarthingInstitute.net*.

Saunas

Saunas use infrared energy to heat your body so that you sweat and eliminate toxins. Sweating is a great way to increase your energy because toxins are a principal cause of low energy in most of us today. At-home infrared saunas can be purchased from $150 to $3,000. For more information on a relatively inexpensive, but effective home sauna, check out the Momentum 98 Company at: *Momentum98.com*.

Bioenergetic Treatments for Pain

Do you experience pain somewhere in your body? If so, you are not alone. According to the American Academy of Pain Medicine (*PainMed.org*), approximately 100 million people in the United States (at least 30 percent of the population) suffer from pain of some type, in the muscles, joints and/or nerves.

Maybe your pain is the result of an injury, stress, illness or nutritional deficiency. Whatever its cause, and whether the pain is acute (short-term) or chronic, chances are bioenergetic medicine can alleviate it, either temporarily or permanently. What's more, it is often effective when other treatments, such as pharmaceutical and natural painkillers, massage, chiropractic, Rolfing and others, are not.

No matter the cause of your pain, bioenergetic medicine provides some excellent and safe alternatives to drugs and other therapies. And unlike drugs, it can often help to heal your body and remove the underlying cause of your pain, rather than just temporarily alleviate your symptoms.

CHAPTER NINETEEN

PEMF Therapy for Pain

In addition to its usefulness for increasing energy and eliminating fatigue, PEMF therapy is also very effective for relieving pain. In fact, PEMF technology devices are probably most famous for their exceptional ability to provide pain relief.

Many other studies have been done which demonstrate the effectiveness of PEMF therapy for reducing pain. Those studies can be found on popular medical research databases such as *PubMed.gov*, as well as at *PEMF.us* and *PEMF.com*.

They do this by reducing inflammation that leads to pain and increasing blood flow and oxygenation to the tissues. The more powerful devices can even repair damaged tissue, including bones! Unlike some forms of pain treatment, which only temporarily relieve symptoms, PEMF therapy can permanently resolve pain by healing damaged tissues and lowering swelling and inflammation.

In the previous section, *Bioenergetic Treatments for Fatigue,* we described PEMF technology at length. For more information on the basics of PEMF therapy and the types of devices that you can purchase for at-home use, please refer back to that section.

The effectiveness of PEMF for tissue healing and regeneration depends upon the type of device, waveform of the electromagnetic pulse and frequencies that you use, as well as the specific condition that you are treating. You may need sophisticated equipment that utilizes very specific frequencies and waveforms and which has the ability to deliver a stronger magnetic field if you have a broken bone or need to regenerate deeply damaged tissues.

According to Dr. Cowden, the sine wave is the least effective form of waveform used for PEMF devices, and the most effective are the "rapid rise, ramp-down" waveform and the "square-wave" waveform. So when you are searching for a PEMF device to purchase, or researching practitioners that use them, it may be helpful to ask the practitioner with the device, or the person selling the device, what kind of waveform their devices use.

PEMF.us provides information on some of the more expensive and sophisticated devices. Some of the cheaper devices that utilize a less powerful magnetic field and lower frequencies are listed in the *Bioenergetic Treatments for Fatigue* section of this book.

Transcutaneous Electrical Nerve Stimulator (TENS) devices, which are commonly prescribed in conventional medicine for pain, utilize a simple square waveform. You can purchase TENS devices for at-home use, and these are often effective for reducing pain and inflammation, but they may or may not regenerate tissue or produce ongoing benefit.

The nervous system often stops responding to the square waveform of a TENS device after several minutes to an hour of continuous use, because it recognizes the square wave as not being "self," so you should use a TENS device for less than an hour at a time, and take a break of several hours between treatments.

PEMF therapy is excellent for alleviating pain in a variety of conditions. For instance, one 2013 study, published in *Rheumatology International,* revealed PEMF to relieve osteoarthritis pain in thirty-four people with knee injuries.

Another study, published in 2012 in the *International Journal of Rheumatic Diseases,* showed PEMF therapy to be an effective method for treating lumbar radiculopathy (which is dysfunction and pain in the nerve branches that come out of the spine in the lower back caused by bulging lumbar discs pressing on those nerves).

In addition to improving lower back pain symptoms, PEMF therapy also seems to be effective for reducing pain caused by compressed nerves. A 2014 study on diabetic rats, published in *Bioelectromagnetics,* revealed PEMFs to help heal diabetic wounds, since PEMFs help the body to create collagen for repairing the wound.

Many other studies have been done which demonstrate the effectiveness of PEMF therapy for reducing pain. Those studies can be found on popular medical research databases such as *PubMed.gov,* as well as at *PEMF.us* and *PEMF.com.*

Because there are a lot of PEMF devices on the market, we recommend that you do some research before purchasing one, and as we previously mentioned, work with a healthcare practitioner that is skilled and knowledgeable about the different types of devices. We recommend contacting PEMF vendors for practitioner referrals, since there is no official database of practitioners that use this type of therapy.

CHAPTER TWENTY

TKM for Pain

We described the basics of The King Method (TKM) in the *Bioenergetic Treatments for Fatigue* section of this book. Incidentally, TKM also has some excellent, inexpensive, do-it-yourself pain reduction sequences.

Here, we will describe a couple of those sequences, which you can do at home, in just 10-30 minutes daily. Although there are at least several

TKM sequences address all kinds of pain, from headaches and sinus pain to knee pain and backaches. We encourage you to contact The King Institute for more information on these sequences, to find one that would best match your particular condition.

TKM doesn't just alleviate symptoms—it can fully resolve even the most serious of health conditions, when the proper sequences are used for the right amount of time. Many testimonials proving the effectiveness of TKM for a variety of conditions can be found at: *KingInstitute.org/services/testimonials.html* types of pain sequences used in TKM, here we provide just two examples. If the sequences that we describe here don't apply to the type of pain that you have, there are others that you can learn to do by purchasing supplemental learning materials at the TKM website: *TheKingInstitute.org.*

The King Institute sells books and DVDs that teach you how to do TKM sequences for all kinds of pain (as well as many other ailments). You can do some of these sequences by yourself, while others will require the help of a partner. Or, if you want to learn how to use TKM to treat more serious health conditions, you can take an online or in-person course through the King Institute.

You may find that doing the sequences once will permanently relieve your pain, especially if that pain is acute or you haven't had it for a long time. For chronic pain, however, you may need to do the sequences periodically or up to one to three times daily for a period of weeks or months. Over time, however, these sequences can permanently relieve many types of pain.

In 1990, I had a 65-year-old male patient who was in a wheelchair, grimacing from excruciating pain. He had ankylosing spondylitis, which is a severe form of arthritis that affects the spine and which can cause it to become fused in a fixed, immobile position. He had urinary and fecal incontinence, and his conventional medical doctors had told him that he would be incontinent his entire life, because the muscles of his rectum and bladder wouldn't contract properly. They also told him that he would have chronic pain in his back and legs for the rest of his life and would have to take narcotics for the pain.

I recommended that he do TKM, and a few months later, he came back into my office, walking with a cane, a smile on his face. He said to me, "I no longer have pain or stool incontinence, and I can tell when I have to catheterize myself." He attributed all these changes in his well-being to TKM! It really made me a believer in the therapy.   —Dr. Lee Cowden

Dr. King's sequences address all kinds of pain, from headaches and sinus pain to knee pain and backaches. We encourage you to contact the King Institute for more information on these sequences, to find one that would best match your particular condition.

Sometimes pain is caused partly by a magnesium deficiency. The United States Department of Agriculture (USDA) website (ars.usda.gov) estimates that only 24 percent of women in the US meet the official US recommended daily allowance (RDA) for magnesium.

In the meantime, following are two examples of Dr. King's pain sequences, to give you an example and better idea of how the sequences work. Dr. King calls this first sequence the R&R 4th stratum. It doesn't take a lot of time to do, and is a powerful treatment for some types of lower back and hip pain, as well as sacrum issues. It can also alleviate neck pain to some degree, depending on the cause of the neck pain.

As all TKM sequences, it can also help to heal other problems that are associated with the energy pathways affected by each particular sequence. So for instance, this sequence can also help to heal bladder and kidney disease, improve your digestion and alleviate fluid retention problems such as edema. It can also resolve feelings of fear (since the emotion of fear has been found to be stored in the kidneys).

In the diagram on the following page, the words "left" and "right" refer to the left and right hands, when they are listed under "Procedures for the Hands." They refer to the left and right sides of the body when listed under "Positions on Body." The numbers that are listed under "Positions on the Body" correspond with the numbers in the diagram.

So, for instance, to do this sequence, you would interpret the top line, which reads "Step 1 right to left 2" as: "Take your right hand and place it on the left side of your body at position 2 (the lower left back, as indicated by the diagram)." You would then place the pads of your right index, middle and ring fingers on the area on your back which corresponds to the number 2 in the diagram, and which, in this case, is on the left side of your body.

Leave your right hand there for the duration of this sequence. At the same time, for steps 2 to 5, take the pads of your left index, middle and ring fingers, and place them sequentially on the different numbered locations, most of which correspond to the left side of your body (and as indicated by the diagram).

Sequence for Revitalizing and Redirecting the Energy of Fourth Stratum.

The diagram illustrates Left sequence Energy Spheres only. Refer to Figure G-4.
LEFT Sequence, sit on the **Right side** of the body.

Procedures For Hands	(to)	Positions On Body E.S.'s
step 1 right	to	left 2
and left	to	right High-1
step 2 left	to	left 4
step 3 left	to	left 12
step 4 left	to	left 11
step 5 left	to	left 23

RIGHT Seq. BE on Left side.

1	L - R	2
	R - L	High-1
2	R - R	4
3	R - R	12
4	R - R	11
5	R - R	23

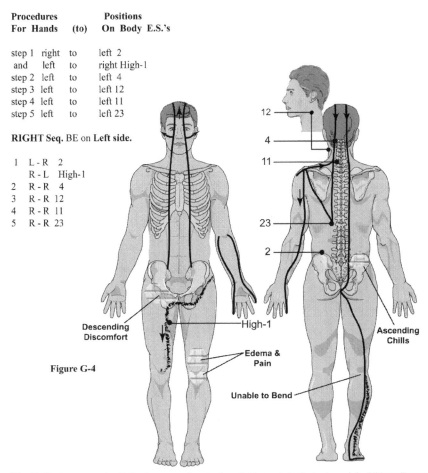

Descending Discomfort

High-1

Ascending Chills

Edema & Pain

Unable to Bend

Figure G-4

The 4th Stratum energy is vital to the proper functioning of all **muscle** in the body, and the **Kidney Energy** and **Bladder Energy**. Its **Ascending** and **Descending energy** helps the **ears** and the emotion of **fear.**

The Stratum color is **Blue**
The tone or musical note correlation is **F**
The emotion is **Fear/Lack**
The Energy Sphere relation is **#23**
The related finger or digit is **Index**

Leave your left hand on each location for about four to five minutes, before moving to the next one. Remember, you'll want to leave your right hand at location number 2 (the lower left back) throughout the duration of the sequence.

So for the first part of this sequence, you'll have your right hand on your lower left back, and your left hand near the top of your right thigh ("High" in this diagram means high on the thigh). Keep your hands in these locations for 4-5 minutes then move your left hand to the next numbered location in the sequence.

The entire sequence should take you about 20 minutes to do. If you do it once or twice daily, chances are, your pain will lessen, and over time, perhaps even fully resolve. If you need more immediate and thorough help, you can either hold each of the locations longer, until you feel relief, or re-apply the entire sequence again, holding each location for approximately 20 minutes or until you experience relief. If you hold each location long enough, your pain will lessen, no matter how severe or acute it is.

As we previously mentioned, TKM doesn't just alleviate symptoms—it can fully resolve even the most serious of health conditions, when the proper sequences are used for the right amount of time. Many testimonials proving the effectiveness of TKM for a variety of conditions can be found at:

KingInstitute.org/services/testimonials.html

While doing TKM, it's also important that you minimize your exposure to electromagnetic fields as much as possible (and even consider removing any metal objects from your body, such as underwire bras, watches, belts or glasses), as these block energy pathways in your body and conduct with electromagnetic fields from the environment, which can disrupt your body's energetic responses to TKM.

Dr. Cowden has found that taking magnesium, L-glutathione, homeopathic and/or herbal detoxification and certain other remedies can amplify the benefits of the TKM pain sequences.

If you suffer from pain, chances are your body doesn't make enough L-glutathione to quench the free radicals that contribute to the pain. For this reason, it can be beneficial to take a liposomal glutathione supplement, either orally or as a cream, while doing TKM.

Sometimes pain is caused partly by a magnesium deficiency. The United States Department of Agriculture (USDA) website (www.ars.usda.gov) estimates that only 24 percent of women in the US meet the official US recommended daily allowance (RDA) for magnesium (and the RDA standards are often quite lax!), so if you have pain, it's also a good idea to take some magnesium on a regular basis. Magnesium dilates the blood vessels and brings more oxygen into oxygen-starved tissues, thereby helping to alleviate the pain.

Below, Dr. Cowden has modified one of Dr. King's pain sequences to include the use of homeopathic-like remedies, which he has also found to enhance the pain-relieving effects of the TKM sequences.

According to Dr. Cowden, the following sequence can be used to relieve symptoms of pain resulting from a wide variety of conditions.

TKM Therapy for Pain Self-Treatment
Modified from Glenn King – *KingInstitute.org*

For this sequence, enlist the help of an assistant. Both you and your assistant should remove all metal objects from your body, including jewelry, wire-rimmed glasses, underwire bras, watches, metal belt buckles, etc. This is because metals disrupt your body's energy flow, and can make the sequence less effective.

Spray some Bliss in a Bottle, which is a natural pain reliever from *SuperGoodStuff.com* into your mouth, as well as onto your pain areas.

Swallow or rub about ¼ to ½ teaspoon of liposomal glutathione anywhere on your skin. We recommend a high-quality glutathione product such as ReadiSorb (*ReadiSorb.com*) or Lipo-Spheric GSH (*LivonLabs.com*).

Take a Magnesium Malate capsule (from NutraMedix or other pharmaceutical-grade supplement company) and hold the powder under your tongue for two minutes before swallowing.

Chase the magnesium down with NutraMedix Burbur Detox (or NutraMedix Parsley Detox) along with eight drops of NutraMedix Pinella in a glass of water.

Alternatively, drink some water containing 10 drops of each of the following: BioActive Nutritionals' Viscum Force, Hepatotox, Lymph II and Nephroplex. These products can be obtained at: *BioactiveNutritional.com*.

Lie on your back on a bed or treatment table with your head at the foot of the bed or table, and have your assistant sit in a chair near the foot of the bed or table.

Begin synchronizing your breathing with that of your assistant. Place the fingers of both hands on your lower anterior rib margins, (this is right where your abdomen joins your ribs just beneath your breasts).

Your seated assistant should put his or her fingers on both sides of your forehead. Hold your fingers in these places until you both feel energetic pulses strongly in your fingers—this should occur after about five minutes. As you do this, only the pads of your index, middle, and ring fingers (and those of your assistant)—from the middle joint of each finger down to near the fingertip—should be touching your body.

After you and your assistant have felt a pulsing sensation in your fingers (in all 4 hands) for at least one full minute, you should then move your fingers to the groin creases on either side of your groin (where your thighs join the pelvic area of your torso).

Your assistant should move his or her chair beside the bed and place the hand that is closest to your head onto the bottom of your breastbone, and his or her other hand onto your midline pubic bone (a few inches below your belly button).

Hold these positions until you both once again feel energetic pulses strongly for at least one minute, which should occur again after about five or more minutes.

Next, position yourself with your head at the top of the bed or table, but remain lying on your back. Then, place the fingers of your right hand on your forehead and the fingers of your left hand on the back of your head, at the junction with your neck.

At the same time, your assistant should place both of their hands under your calves, with fingers held together (not spread apart) and fingertips near the skin crease behind your knee where your calf joins your thigh.

Place pillows under your arms during this process so that your arms don't get tired and can be as relaxed as possible. You and your assistant should leave your hands on these TKM points for about 10 to 15 minutes.

After you have completed steps 1 through 8, assess your pain level. If it has gone down some but not enough, repeat steps 2 through 8 again. The entire sequence (steps 2 through 8) should take you about 25 to 35 minutes each time that you do the full sequence, depending upon your body's response to the sequence, as well as your pain level.

CHAPTER TWENTY-ONE

Low-Level (Cold) Laser Therapy (LLLT)

The low-level laser therapy (LLLT) device is another great, inexpensive, do-it-yourself tool that we highly recommend for alleviating many types of pain. LLLT consists of coherent (or focused, rather than dispersed) light with wavelengths that are usually in the red and/or infra-red part of the electromagnetic spectrum. This type of light is profoundly healing to the body.

> **LLLT is a great therapy that you can do at home or while traveling, if you need quick, safe, cheap and non-invasive pain relief.**

The light is usually transmitted through a small device that utilizes low-level lasers, with or without additional red or infrared non-coherent light-emitting diodes. For this therapy, you simply place the laser over the places on your body where you have pain, and then slowly move it around those areas.

Many studies show that LLLT is effective for relieving acute or short-term pain in a variety of pain conditions, including temporomandibular joint disorder (TMJ), or jaw joint pain, rheumatoid and osteoarthritis; acute and chronic neck pain, tendonitis, and chronic joint disorders. It may also be useful for relieving lower back, shoulder and other types of pain.

For instance, one study, published in 2014 in *Lasers in Medical Science* showed LLLT to relieve pain in thirty-three people with osteoarthritis.

Another study, published in 2014 in this same journal, revealed LLLT to be effective for relieving symptoms of temporomandibular joint disorder (TMJ), or pain and stiffness in the jaw.

Many other similar studies on LLLT and its effects on different types of pain can be found on the research database: *PubMed.gov.*

LLLT devices vary in their intensity and ability to penetrate the body. Little red low-intensity lasers, which you can purchase at an office supply store, are useful for treating pain in the finger and toe joints. These emit 0.5 mW of energy.

Higher-powered non-pulsed class III lasers can emit anywhere from 5 to 500 mW of power, and are useful for treating pain elsewhere in the body. In general, the higher intensity lasers have the deepest penetration into the tissues. For instance, research has shown that 600 to 1000 nanometer wavelength (red to near infrared) lasers have the best penetration into the tissues, along with the greatest effects upon cellular energy production and inflammation.

LLLT devices that utilize about 1000 nm wavelengths have been shown to improve brain function in people with dementia, but red LLLT devices, which utilize a wavelength of about 650 nm, appear to be more helpful for re-growing hair and reducing the appearance of wrinkles. But even the lower powered lasers can actually be used to re-grow hair and reduce the appearance of wrinkles.

Correspondingly, LLLT therapy devices can cost anywhere from several hundred to several thousand dollars, depending on the device's intensity and quality, and whether it is programmable and allows you to modulate the frequencies.

Some LLLT devices, though, are very inexpensive. For instance, you can purchase ten of the 100 mW red lasers for about $150 or one red laser for about $30, from *LuckLaser.com*. Such lasers can be effective for reducing inflammation and pain in the small joints.

Low-level lasers, if used properly, are relatively safe and without side effects, but you need to be extremely careful to never shine a laser into your eyes, because you can blind yourself by doing this, if the period of exposure is long enough.

If you are using a laser that has less than 100 mW of power, you can move it slowly over your pain area for up to 30 minutes, without having to worry about experiencing any negative side effects. The higher the wattage that the laser delivers, the less time that you can use it on an area, without burning the tissue. Also, the smaller the area that is "painted" with the laser, the less time it can be used before burns occur.

We recommend that you start by treating any pain area for only 5 to 10 minutes at a time, since less laser treatment is often better than more. If the laser doesn't successfully reduce your pain after an initial treatment, you might incrementally increase the treatment time by five minutes every 12 to 24 hours. We recommend not holding higher-powered lasers over the same skin location for too long, as these can potentially burn or damage your tissues.

If placing the laser over the pain location doesn't relieve your discomfort, try placing the laser somewhere along the acupuncture meridian on your body that corresponds with the pain location.

To determine where the meridian lines are on your body, simply look up "Chinese meridian chart" on the Internet, to find diagrams that will show you the locations of the meridians, and then pick a point along the same meridian where you also have pain, and shine the laser on that area.

The charts are fairly simple and straightforward to read. You can also look up what are called Chinese or Nogier auriculotherapy charts and shine your laser for a few seconds on the meridian points on your ears that correspond with the pain locations on your body.

LLLT is a great therapy that you can do at home or while traveling, if you need quick, safe, cheap and non-invasive pain relief. This therapy may be less powerful than, for example, PEMF therapy, and therefore may not be the best choice for you if your pain is severe, but we recommend trying it before pain medications, which almost always damage the body in some way. It is also an ideal alternative to chiropractic or massage therapy, which can get expensive and time-consuming if your pain is chronic, and often provides only temporary pain relief.

Low-level lasers can be purchased at a variety of online retailers, such as Quantum Healing Lasers: *Quantum-Healing-Lasers.com/*.

CHAPTER TWENTY-TWO

Other Pain Therapies

The pain therapies and devices that we mention in this section are really only the tip of the proverbial iceberg, as there are many other pain devices and energetic healing modalities for pain reduction that you can do or use. We simply recommend those that Dr. Cowden has found to be most helpful for his patients, and which we both have found to have a substantial amount of anecdotal evidence or research to back their effectiveness.

Following we list a few other tools that have been scientifically proven to be helpful for pain reduction. You may want to look into doing some of these, if you find that the other therapies in this section don't suit you.

Acupuncture

We described the basics of acupuncture and how it works in the *Bioenergetic Treatments for Fatigue* section of this book. Please refer to this section for more information on why acupuncture is such a great treatment for low energy, pain and other common health conditions.

One meta-analysis of 29 studies, the results of which were published in the October 2012 *Archives of Internal Medicine,* revealed acupuncture to be effective for relieving pain in a variety of conditions about 50 percent of the time.

Acupuncture reduces or eliminates pain via several means: first, by stimulating blood flow and increasing oxygen to the tissues; second, by lowering inflammation; and third, by improving detoxification of the tissues.

It has substantial research to back its effectiveness. For instance, one meta-analysis of 29 studies, the results of which were published in the October 2012 *Archives of Internal Medicine,* revealed acupuncture to be effective for relieving pain in a variety of conditions about 50 percent of the time.

The analysis involved more than 28,000 patients with all types of pain conditions. The studies showed acupuncture to be most effective for treating low back and neck pain, menstrual cramps, osteoarthritis, knee pain, myofascial pain, and postoperative dental pain. It was also sometimes effective for other pain conditions, such as fibromyalgia and tennis elbow, as well as for migraines and other types of headaches.

However, more research is needed to determine the usefulness of acupuncture for other types of pain conditions. Given these outcomes though, we suggest giving acupuncture a try if you suffer from pain of any kind, especially those types of pain for which it has proven to be most effective.

IONTOPHORESIS

Iontophoresis is a great therapy to try if you have pain caused by foci infections, or localized pockets of infection in your body. Environmental toxins also tend to reside in these areas.

The therapy involves passing an electrical current through the front side of your body to the backside of your body using electrode pads, which are placed on your skin on either side of your body.

The electrode pads are moistened with a charged chemical substance, usually some type of anti-inflammatory medication, a toxin binder or bioactive agent. An electrical current carries the chemical molecules from one pad, through your body, to the other pad.

The toxin-binding agents used in iontophoresis have the ability to bind with whatever they contact as they move through your body. This means that they can bind to heavy metals or other toxins, which are then carried through your body, then through your skin, to the other pad.

As toxins get removed from your tissues, it results in better functioning of those tissues and less irritation of the nerves in those tissues by any remaining toxins. Inotophoresis can, therefore, be a fantastic way to not only eliminate focal toxins, but also lower pain-causing inflammation from those toxins. Practitioners who have an iontophoresis device and who perform this procedure can probably best be found at The Klinghardt Academy website: *KlinghardtAcademy.com.*

INFRARED PHOTONIC FOCAL DETOXIFICATION

Sometimes pain is caused by an accumulation of environmental toxins in different parts of the body. Or, toxins tend to accumulate in already damaged or injured tissue, which then worsens the initial pain condition.

To find practitioners that do infrared photonic focal detoxification and Laser Energetic Detox, visit the Academy for Comprehensive Integrative Medicine website: *ACIMConnect.com/Resources* **Click on** *FindHealthProfessional.aspx.*

Another strategy in bioenergetic medicine for removing these toxins, and thereby the pain, is called infrared photonic focal detox. This involves putting a homeopathic homaccord (the harmonic energetic signature) of a toxin into a clear-glass vial filled with water and minerals, or water and ethanol, and then shining an infrared light through that vial, onto the location of your body where you hurt, for several minutes at a time.

As you do this, you will energetically "shake loose" from that area any toxins, which your body will then eliminate. This type of therapy is also exceptionally useful for treating toxic foci, which are areas of concentrated infection or toxins in the body. Some common foci areas in the body include: wisdom teeth extraction sites, root canal sites, the sinuses, gallbladder, appendix, fallopian tubes and the prostate.

While the concept of this therapy is simple, it is best to not attempt to do it yourself, but instead, enlist the help of a trained healthcare practitioner, as you can have a severe detoxification reaction that then might require managed detoxification support.

Any practitioner that is knowledgeable about electrodermal screening can learn how to do this treatment by taking a one-hour laser detoxification course from the Academy for Comprehensive Integrative Medicine: *ACIMConnect.com*. To find practitioners that do infrared photonic focal detoxification and Laser Energetic Detox, visit the Academy for Comprehensive Integrative Medicine website: *ACIMConnect.com/Resources/FindHealthProfessional.aspx*

Bioenergetic Treatments for Insomnia

Many of us in today's hectic, toxic world don't sleep well; we sleep fitfully, or don't get in enough hours. Maybe you awaken in the morning feeling a tad sluggish or tired, or perhaps are downright exhausted, due to an inadequate amount or poor quality of sleep.

The Clear Mind website also has a link to studies which show the Clear Mind System to have an 80 percent success rate at reducing or eliminating symptoms of insomnia (as well as other neurological conditions).

Many factors contribute to insomnia and restless sleep. These include: emotional and mental stress; hormone and neurotransmitter imbalances; certain diseases and exposure to environmental toxins; prescription sleep medications (which make sleep problems worse over the long run); geopathic stress and electromagnetic fields from cell phones, power lines, etc.—just to name a few!

Electromagnetic pollution may be an especially pervasive cause of insomnia nowadays, unbeknownst to many of us. As we previously mentioned, we are living in a sea of electromagnetic fields, which come from cell phone towers, power lines, smart meters, Wi-Fi and poor wiring in the home. These fields disrupt the body's electromagnetic energy and, over time, can cause a myriad of health problems, including insomnia.

It is important to eliminate electromagnetic and geopathic pollution from your environment as much as possible if you suspect that these are contributing to your insomnia. Treatments for insomnia, such as bioenergetic devices, herbs, drugs and the like, may not be effective until you are able to remove or mitigate the effects of EMF and geopathic stress from your environment.

In the first book in this series, *Create a Toxin-Free Body & Home ... Starting Today*, we describe ways that you can protect your body from EMF pollution. It is important to protect your body as much as you can from these fields, and at the same time do whatever you can to get your energetic field re-balanced. Great ways to do this are with PEMF technology, TKM or acupuncture, which we described in previous sections of this book.

Other therapies such as biofeedback devices, which affect brain wave patterns, are another fantastic option for restoring sleep. These devices aren't intended to balance your body's energy, but instead, utilize energy to manipulate your brain wave patterns and put your body into a state of rest, so that you can sleep.

In the following chapters, we describe light and sound machines, biofeedback devices, and homeopathic or energetically imprinted herbal remedies, as well as other powerful bioenergetic modalities for healing from insomnia and restless sleep, no matter the cause.

> **Neurofeedback devices are a type of biofeedback device that measures your brain waves, and then uses that information to produce a signal that can be used as feedback to regulate your brain activity. It is an extraordinarily useful bioenergetic medicine tool that can improve symptoms of insomnia in most people.**

CHAPTER TWENTY-THREE

Biofeedback Devices

Biofeedback therapy utilizes electromagnetic instruments to provide information on different physiological functions of your body, with the goal of being able to manipulate those functions. Some of the processes that can be positively controlled and altered to facilitate healing include: the brain waves, heart rate, skin temperature and pain perception, among others.

Neurofeedback devices are a type of biofeedback device that specifically measures your brain waves, and then uses that information to produce a signal that can be used as feedback to regulate your brain activity. It is an extraordinarily useful bio-energetic medicine tool that can fully resolve or at least improve symptoms of insomnia in most people.

Unlike dangerous chemical sleep medications, such as benzodiazepenes (sedatives), antidepressants and other drugs, which are often given in conventional medicine to treat insomnia, neurofeedback doesn't cause addictions or toxicity in the liver, or create long-term neurotransmitter imbalances or other undesirable side effects. Instead, it entrains your brain, or essentially teaches it, how to behave like it's supposed to at night! Over time, it can permanently alter your brain wave patterns and positively affect your brain's chemistry.

The light and sound machine is another type of brain entrainment device that helps to restore proper brain wave patterns so that your brain knows to shut down at night.

Many studies have proven neurofeedback to have a strong track record of success at treating a variety of neurological conditions, not just insomnia. For instance, it has proven to be useful for reducing symptoms of autism, epilepsy, headaches, depression, anxiety and brain damage from strokes.

Many of us have had a head and/or brain injury sometime during our lives, but may or may not be aware of it. For instance, we may have had a prolonged or difficult birth, which damaged our brain in some way, unbeknownst to us. Quantitative EEG mapping tests have also proven that some viruses, microbes and toxins can cause brain damage patterns similar to those of physical traumas, such as when a person is dealt a blunt blow to the head.

Brain injuries can contribute to symptoms of insomnia, as well as anxiety, depression, impaired concentration and/or memory; difficulty with problem solving, and other neurological issues. Neurofeedback is excellent for repairing such damage, and thereby mitigating symptoms.

Like PEMF therapy, neurofeedback can be done in a clinic, but some companies sell neurofeedback devices that you can use at home. These devices often have sensors that you place on different locations on your head, and which are used to provide feedback to the device about your brain wave patterns. The device then uses this feedback as input to normalize those patterns, and subsequently, your brain function, so that you can sleep when you are supposed to sleep, and remain awake when you are supposed to be awake.

One type of neurofeedback system that has a strong track record of success is called Clear Mind. According to the Clear Mind Center website: *ClearMindCenter.com*, "Clear Mind uses electroencephalography (EEG) to provide a signal that can be used by a person to receive feedback about brain activity. The EEG signal is fed into computer software first, then the feedback, usually a movie or music, is returned to the person being trained.

This feedback loop can produce changes in brain wave activity. The process used to adjust brain wave activity is known as operant conditioning, which is a method whereby rewards for positive behavior increase learning capabilities.

According to the Clear Mind website, for the clinical version of Clear Mind, a computer monitors your brain waves while you watch a movie or listen to music. For the home version, you simply wear a pair of glasses with blinking lights, while four sensors provide input on your brain wave patterns back to the device.

Whenever your brain shows deviations from normal brain wave activity, the computer triggers an audio or visual cue that alerts your brain that you are outside of the normal ranges. The brain then subconsciously adjusts itself back to a normal pattern. When this process is repeated long enough, the brain learns to stay within the normal ranges on its own without the help of the device. As your brain function normalizes, your symptoms begin to disappear!

The Clear Mind website also has a link to studies which show the Clear Mind System to have an 80 percent success rate at reducing or eliminating symptoms of insomnia (as well as other neurological conditions).

> I suffered from severe insomnia for years, and often relied upon sleep medication to get to sleep. After awhile, the sleep medication caused my insomnia to worsen, so I began doing Clear Mind therapy. This therapy not only helped me to wean off of the sleep medication, which I had been addicted to for a long time, but effectively helped me to sleep again. I had to do other therapies as well to fully resolve the insomnia, such as replenishing my body with amino acids such as 5-HTP and doing bioidentical hormone replacement, but the Clear Mind device was instrumental in helping me to be free from this debilitating symptom. —Connie Strasheim

Clear Mind sessions at a clinic might cost $100 to $200 per session. At the time of the writing of this book, a personal device for at-home use, called the "Neurointegrator," was available for approximately $3500. Severe cases of insomnia and other conditions may require 50 or more daily treatments, so it can be worthwhile to invest in a home unit, rather than go to a clinic that offers treatments.

The home device isn't as fine-tuned as the clinical version of Clear Mind, but it is usually effective enough for treating generalized depression, anxiety and insomnia. More complicated neurological disorders, such as autism and Post-Traumatic Stress Disorder (PTSD), however, may respond better to professional Clear Mind treatments, which can only be done at a healthcare practitioner's office. For more information on Clear Mind, or to find a practitioner in your area that does Clear Mind, check out the Clear Mind website: *ClearMindCenter.com.*

CHAPTER TWENTY-FOUR

Light and Sound Machines

The light and sound machine is another type of brain entrainment device that helps to restore proper brain wave patterns, so that your brain knows to shut down at night. It "feeds" fixed energetic frequencies to your brain, rather than utilizing feedback from your brain to adjust your brainwave frequencies.

One advantage of light and sound machines is that they are relatively affordable, compared to some other types of therapies. You can purchase a good light and sound machine for anywhere from $159 to $600 on websites such as *ToolsForWellness.com*.

Therefore, it utilizes pre-programmed brain wave pattern protocols to deliver frequencies to your brain. It does this with the aid of blinking-light glasses, and/or audio sounds which are delivered through a set of headphones. With these frequencies, the light and sound machine gradually entrains your brain into a slow delta-wave pattern, which your body needs for deep sleep.

Of the many therapies that I have used on my patients over the years, I have found the light and sound machine to be one of the best for insomnia. Some people prefer to use only the sound component of the device for sleep, while others prefer to use only the light component. Fortunately, both of these can be effective by themselves, although it's preferable to use both the sound and light components together for best results.   —Dr. Lee Cowden

Most of these types of devices start by entraining your brain at a higher frequency, and then slowly lowering that frequency until your brain effectively reaches a delta frequency, at which time you are completely asleep!

So, for instance, the device might start by entraining your brain at a beta frequency of around 30 Hz. Your brain is in a beta state when you are fully awake and alert. Over a few minutes, the device will slowly ramp down the frequencies into the alpha range, say, 8 to 13 Hz. The alpha state puts your brain into a more relaxed state. Then, the device will ramp the frequencies down even further, into the theta range, say 5 to 7 Hz, and finish the program in the delta frequency range, which is about 1 to 4 Hz.

By the time you get down into the 1 to 4 Hz range, you are asleep, whether you want to be or not! Both the flashing lights on the glasses and the audio sounds function to slowly entrain your brain down into this delta wave pattern.

One advantage of light and sound machines is that they are relatively affordable, compared to some other types of therapies. You can purchase a good light and sound machine for anywhere from $159 to $600 on websites such as *ToolsForWellness.com*.

CHAPTER TWENTY-FIVE

Homeopathic and Energetically Imprinted Remedies

Homeopathic and other energetic remedies are useful for treating a wide variety of conditions, including insomnia, and provide a gentle way to alleviate symptoms, when other tools might prove to be either too expensive or harsh on the body.

Homeopathic remedies are generally safe and non-toxic, so if your time or finances are limited, you could try using one or more of the remedies on your own, before consulting with a healthcare practitioner.

The general principles of homeopathy and energetically imprinted herbal remedies will be described later in this book, in the section on *Bioenergetic Treatments for Anxiety,* so please refer to that section for basic information about what they are and how they work.

Light and sound devices are powerful for inducing sleep, but may not be affordable and can be too time-consuming for some people. Also, the flashing lights can trigger seizures in people who are prone to seizures. A few others may be so sensitive to electromagnetic fields that they cannot even tolerate battery-operated light and sound machines (although this is relatively rare).

According to the Centers for Disease Control, it is estimated that least one in ten people in the United States will develop depression or anxiety, or both, sometime during their lifetime.

For this reason, we also recommend homeopathic and energetic remedies as alternatives to these therapies, since they are gentle, inexpensive and don't require much of an investment of time. Also, homeopathic remedies can sometimes be targeted, or tailored, to the specific cause of your insomnia.

We recommend that you choose a homeopathic remedy based on the characteristics and type of insomnia that you have, as well as your personal constitution and history. There are a wide variety of remedies to choose from, and you may find it most useful to work with a homeopath or other holistic doctor experienced in their use, to determine the one(s) that would best fit you.

You can get insights into the remedy or remedies that might be most adequate for you and your particular situation by reading homeopath David Curtin's article, "Sleep Problems" featured on the British Homeopathic Association webpage: *BritishHomeopathic.org.*

This page contains a list of some commonly used remedies for insomnia and for what circumstances each remedy is indicated. For instance, Nux vomica is a remedy that is useful for people who awaken around 3 a.m., with their brain full of thoughts! Coffea is useful when you are completely sleepless, or if you sleep until 3 a.m. but then are awake or doze the rest of the night. Belladonna is helpful if you have anxious, frightful or vivid dreams. Other remedies described on the webpage include: stramonium, valeriana, pulsatilla and arsenicum, among others.

The Alpha-Stim® device has been found anecdotally, as well as in a couple of research studies, to be effective for inducing sleep.

Homeopathic remedies are generally safe and non-toxic, so if your time or finances are limited, you could try using one or more of the remedies on your own, before consulting with a healthcare practitioner. If that doesn't prove to be an effective strategy, you might then consider working with an experienced homeopath to see if you get better results.

Some great energetically imprinted herbal remedies for sleep include the NutraMedix products Babuna and Amantilla (*NutraMedix.com*), which are energetically imprinted chamomile and valerian root extracts, respectively. Babuna has been found to be especially effective for children, and Amantilla more so for adults. Amantilla is also described in greater detail in the *Bioenergetic Treatments for Anxiety* section of this book.

Both homeopathic and energetic remedies utilize energy to achieve a desired result in the body, though via different means. We encourage you to read the chapter on homeopathy later in this book for more information on the differences between these types of energetic remedies.

CHAPTER TWENTY-SIX

Other Therapies for Insomnia

BIOMAT

According to the Biomat.com website, the Biomat is a therapeutic mat that combines the energy of far infrared rays, negative ions and the conductive properties of amethyst crystals to deliver relaxing, regenerative and deep-penetrating heat to your body.

> We recommend checking out the Biomat as an additional option for resolving sleeplessness, and for maintaining overall wellness. Biomats range from $600 (for a mini-biomat) to $1900 for a full-sized mat.

The technology is based on Nobel prize-winning scientific research pioneered by NASA and is effective for helping to heal the body of a variety of conditions, including insomnia. Among the other benefits of the Biomat, and according to the Biomat site, this therapeutic mat also "repairs damaged tissue, reduces joint and muscle soreness, chronic neck and back pain, toxicity, oxidation levels, inflammation and arthritis, and circulatory issues."

We recommend checking out the Biomat as an additional option for resolving sleeplessness, and for maintaining overall wellness. Biomats range from $600 (for a mini-biomat) to $1900 for a full-sized mat.

PEMF DEVICES

PEMF devices can also be incredibly helpful for resolving sleeplessness, if you use the proper device and frequencies for the right amount of time. The iMRS is one type of PEMF mat that has been proven anecdotally to be effective for some people for this purpose, although other PEMF devices, especially those that we mentioned in the *Bioenergetic Treatments for Fatigue and Pain* sections of this book can be effective as well.

Neurofeedback devices are among the most powerful tools in bioenergetic medicine for healing not only from insomnia, but also depression and other mood disorders. See Chapter 27 for more information.

The frequencies generated by the device put the body into a relaxation state, and calm the nervous system. The iMRS can also be purchased to include a sound and light device and heart rate variability (HRV) sensor, the latter of which helps to fine-tune the frequencies of the device to your body's needs.

If you are sensitive to electromagnetic fields, just a few minutes on a PEMF mat such as the iMRS can be sufficient to bring your body into a deep state of rest. If you spend too many minutes on the mat, however, it can have an opposite effect and over-stimulate your nervous system or cause a strong detoxification reaction.

Treatment times with PEMF technology vary according to your current state of health and unique biochemistry. One person may benefit from a five-minute treatment, while another might need an hour of treatment daily.

When it comes to PEMF devices, and as mentioned earlier in this book, we always recommend starting out slowly, using a low frequency and only for a few minutes daily. Over time, you may obtain better benefit by using the PEMF device for longer periods of time, say, 30 to 60 minutes daily, but we never recommend using a device for this long in the beginning.

If you decide to try PEMF technology for sleep, we recommend that you lie on a PEMF mat or use another comparable device for just a few minutes before bedtime, for several nights in a row. If that doesn't improve your rest, you can try increasing the time by several more minutes, to see if that produces an effect. You will probably have to experiment a bit to find the frequencies that will best work for you, but most people seem to obtain some benefit from PEMF therapy when they use the right device, treatment time and frequencies.

ALPHA-STIM® DEVICES

This device uses cranial electrotherapy to deliver micro-current to your brain, to manipulate its electromagnetic energy. The treatment is delivered through a small electrical device with electrodes that attach to your ears and other parts of your body. Like the light-sound machine, the Alpha-Stim® delivers a sequence of frequencies to your brain, which gradually entrain it into a delta wave state, which induces deep sleep.

The Alpha-Stim® device has been found anecdotally, as well as in a couple of research studies, to be effective for inducing sleep. For more information on this device, we encourage you to visit the Alpha-Stim® website: *Alpha-Stim.com,* which also contains a peer-reviewed analysis of the effects of the device on 2500 patients with insomnia and other neurological disorders.

In Chapter 28, we introduced EVOX, a computerized program developed by the ZYTO Corporation that helps to heal depression caused by traumatic memories, through a process called Perception Reframing, and by delivering to your body energetic frequencies that are embedded in your voice.

If you live in the US, the Alpha-Stim® is only available for purchase via prescription. If you live outside the US, however, you don't need a prescription. Although you must obtain a prescription to purchase it in the US, one of the benefits of this device is that your insurance plan might pay for it. Otherwise, these devices can range in price from $795 to $1195.

The Alpha-Stim® website also contains several testimonials of people who have been healed from insomnia by using the device. For instance, one woman from Texas writes, "I have been using the Alpha-Stim® for six months now for treatment of insomnia and depression. The change in how I feel is amazing. It is like a miracle. I am now on half of the antidepressant (that I take) and I no longer use sleeping aids. No medication has ever treated my insomnia or depression as well as this. Why isn't the Alpha-Stim® out more in the public?"

> I once had a patient in the early 1990s that suffered from severe insomnia and sleepwalking. The police called me early one morning, and said that they had picked her up at a busy street intersection in Dallas at 3 a.m.. She was wearing her pajamas and directing traffic, and was startled when they awakened her. I had just seen her for the first time a few days prior to this event.
>
> Her previous doctor had put her on multiple psychotropic drugs and strong pharmaceutical sleep medications. Her melatonin levels were taken the following day after her police arrest, and found to be essentially zero.
>
> I recommended that she take the amino acid supplement L-tryptophan, and do Alpha-Stim® sessions, while she gradually tapered off of most of her pharmaceutical sleep medications that she had been taking. By doing this, her insomnia and sleepwalking gradually resolved. —Dr. Lee Cowden

Bioenergetic Treatments
for Depression

If you suffer from symptoms of depression, which include not only feelings of deep sadness, hopelessness or discouragement, but also low energy, trouble thinking, pain, insomnia and/or anxiety (basically all of the other conditions we describe in this book!) among others, then know that you're not alone.

According to the Centers for Disease Control, it is estimated that at least one in ten people in the United States will develop depression or anxiety, or both, sometime during their lifetime. The number of people who suffer from depression is probably much higher than that, since a lot of cases of depression go unreported, and many people don't recognize when they are depressed.

Depression can be intermittent, or constant. It can last for weeks, months or years. According to the American Psychological Association, Major Depressive Disorder is the leading cause of disability in the U.S. in people aged 15 to 44.

The incidence of mood disorders in the US and other industrialized nations is rising, due to a variety of factors. First, our food supply is terribly nutrient-depleted, due to modern corporate farming and agricultural practices. This means that our bodies aren't getting the raw materials that they need to create hormones and neurotransmitters, both of which we need for mood stability, proper cognition, energy and restful sleep.

Also, the huge amounts of environmental toxins to which we are exposed daily can directly or indirectly cause depression. Mercury and lead toxicity, for instance, have been implicated in mood disorders. Getting rid of these toxins is just as essential for healing, but can take time.

A 2003 study, published in the French journal Pathologie Biologie also showed that people who live within 300 meters (about 980 feet) from a cellphone tower are much more likely to experience depression and insomnia, so electromagnetic pollution may also contribute to these conditions.

In addition, the fast-paced, isolated lives that many of us live, or the emotional traumas that we carry from the past, can cause depression. When depression is caused by trauma or an unhealthy lifestyle, we recommend healing the emotions behind the depression, with cognitive strategies such as counseling and prayer, and/or the energy psychology treatments that we describe in this section.

> Described in Chapter 28, EVOX recreates new frequency patterns that help you to positively reframe your beliefs and perceptions about life. The EVOX reframing process enables you to see relationships, opportunities, challenges and circumstances in more beneficial ways.

Conventional medical doctors typically treat depression and anxiety with antidepressant medication and sometimes sedatives. These drugs actually damage your body over the long run by depleting its neurotransmitter and neurotransmitter receptor levels. So your condition after having taken a pharmaceutical drug for any prolonged period of time can often be worse than your initial one!

If you see a holistic medical doctor, he or she might have prescribed you amino acids, vitamins, minerals, hormone replacement therapy, and other nutrients to heal and restore your body's chemistry. While these are important and useful, balancing neurotransmitters and hormones is tricky business, as well as expensive, and supplementation doesn't always provide great results for everyone. Plus, it takes time to see results from nutritional supplementation—usually months. So what can you do in the meantime?

Fortunately, bioenergetic medicine offers some lifesaving strategies for healing from depression and other mood disorders, until the other factors that either caused or contributed to your depression (such as trauma or a poor diet) are dealt with. In some cases, you may not have to address the root cause of the depression, as energy psychology strategies will often automatically remove the root cause.

These strategies are safer and often more effective than pharmaceutical drugs, and even amino acid therapy, depending upon the cause of the depression. In the following sections, we describe some of these amazing healing strategies. Be encouraged—there are ways to heal from depression, other than through traditional counseling and drug therapy!

CHAPTER TWENTY-SEVEN

Neurofeedback Devices

Neurofeedback devices are among the most powerful tools in bioenergetic medicine for healing not only from insomnia, but also depression and other mood disorders. They reduce symptoms of depression in the same way that they reduce symptoms of insomnia—by restoring proper brain wave frequency patterns throughout your brain using a device that assesses your brain activity, then providing feedback to your brain so that it self-regulates.

With regular neurofeedback sessions, your brain will begin to function better, and will create new neural networks and pathways to self-regulate, so that over time, it will no longer need the feedback device to work properly.

The Clear Mind therapy, which we described in the previous section on insomnia, is also a great choice for alleviating symptoms of a variety of mood disorders, including depression. The Clear Mind website also provides research studies which prove the effectiveness of neurofeedback for treating depression. For more information on these studies, visit: *ClearMindCenter.com.*

CHAPTER TWENTY-EIGHT

EVOX

EVOX is a computerized program developed by the ZYTO Corporation that helps to heal depression caused by traumatic memories, through a process called Perception Reframing, and by delivering to your body energetic frequencies that are embedded in your voice.

Your thoughts are comprised of energetic frequencies. Some researchers believe that the energy frequencies of positive thoughts are higher than the frequencies of negative thoughts. And scientists have proven that we can affect the expression of our DNA with the energy of our thoughts!

Similarly, your voice contains energetic frequencies that correspond with your perceptions (or beliefs) about your life. EVOX uses the frequencies that are embedded in your voice to analyze your perceptions about different aspects of your life, and then provides energetic feedback to reframe, or recreate, those perceptions.

It works like this. The EVOX records your voice frequencies (not your words) and then creates a software-generated map based on a computer analysis of your voice. Subsequently, it creates a recording containing perception-reframing frequencies (which, as we mentioned, are derived from your own voice frequencies) that are delivered back to your body through a hand-cradle electrode.

At the same time, you listen to pleasant instrumental music, which is played back to you through a set of headphones. Those voice-generated frequencies help to "shake loose" the harmful energetic imprint of traumatic memories that are embedded in all of the cells of your body (and which are called your emotional cellular memory). Therefore, they act as a type of re-programming for your mind and body.

At the same time, EVOX recreates new frequency patterns that help you to positively reframe your beliefs and perceptions about life. The EVOX reframing process enables you to see relationships, opportunities, challenges and circumstances in more beneficial ways.

EVOX is especially useful for healing mood disorders such as depression, because our negative perceptions about life often occur as a result of past trauma, and can negatively impact our current reality, performance and relationships. EVOX helps us to reframe those perceptions.

For instance, someone who might be a good writer, but who was shamed as a child for the stories that he wrote, might consider himself to be a poor writer, even though he is in reality a good writer. The EVOX technology would help him to reframe his perspective about himself, so that it more accurately reflects a truth that isn't colored by past negative experiences.

> The power of EVOX is illustrated by one of my former patients who had several physical health problems and was also the most negative person that you could imagine. She was unhappy in her marriage and had no friends at work. She agreed to do some EVOX sessions.
>
> After the fourth session, she showed up at my office, giggling. She said that she now had new friends at work and felt good. Most of her original symptoms had disappeared. The following day, her husband came to my office and said that he didn't know exactly what we had done to his wife but then said, "Thank you for a new wife. I want to do the therapy that she did."
> —Dr. Lee Cowden

EVOX therapy must be done in a healthcare practitioner's office. Sessions typically cost around $100 to $150. You should experience a noticeable change in your emotions, and possibly even your physical symptoms, after about three sessions. Radical changes often occur after about six sessions.

Like all mind-body therapies, some people will receive more benefit from EVOX therapy than others. Results can range from significant healing of your physical and emotional problems, to small, but noticeable changes in your overall well-being.

To find a practitioner that does EVOX, we recommend doing an Internet search, using the terms "EVOX practitioner" along with your city or state. Due to legal constraints and company policy, ZYTO doesn't provide a list of names and addresses of practitioners that use the technology.

CHAPTER TWENTY-NINE

Emotional Freedom Technique (EFT)

Emotional Freedom Technique (EFT) is an energy psychology healing modality that is based upon the principles of psychotherapy, Thought Field Therapy (TFT), neuro-linguistic programming (NLP), acupressure, and bioenergetic balancing.

EFT is based on the idea that stagnant emotions create an imbalance in your body's meridian system. EFT doesn't aim to cognitively resolve past trauma that can lead to depression, but instead, re-balances the meridians and re-programs positive emotions and beliefs into your cellular memory.

For this therapy, you tap on different acupressure meridian points on your body to release the stagnant energy of negative emotions that are stored there. At the same time, you speak affirmations to counter the problem that is causing your depression.

EFT is based on the idea that stagnant emotions create an imbalance in your body's meridian system. EFT doesn't aim to cognitively resolve past trauma that can lead to depression, but instead, re-balances the meridians and re-programs positive emotions and beliefs into your cellular memory. These two things by themselves are thought to automatically release the negative emotions.

The Founder of EFT, Gary Craig, likens EFT to acupuncture. On his website, *EmoFree.com,* he states that EFT helps to heal emotions in a similar way to how acupuncture heals the physical body. He says,

> EFT breathes fresh air into the healing process by borrowing from the Chinese meridian system. EFT combines the physical benefits of acupuncture with the cognitive benefits of conventional psychotherapy for a much faster, more complete treatment of emotional issues, and the physical and performance issues that often result.

The affirmative statements that you speak during EFT always involve first verbally acknowledging the most prominent negative emotion that you have—whether it is fear, worry, sadness, anger, rejection, or so on—while tapping on the appropriate acupressure, or meridian point. Then, you follow this with a positive affirmation or life-giving statement that is designed to replace the old, limiting, disease-causing belief that led to your negative emotions, while still tapping on the same acupressure point.

The tapping involved in EFT apparently functions to balance the meridians, while the affirmations involved in EFT help to remove negative emotions that are embedded in the cellular memory of the body. To achieve the most benefit from EFT, it is important that you uncover the underlying issue that is causing your depression, in order to fully release and clear the emotions of that issue from your body.

> REMAP interventions are able to anesthetize the intense emotions behind an upsetting memory. So, just as you would be given an anesthetic before undergoing a painful surgery, so REMAP provides an anesthesia of sorts while you undergo the process of emotional healing.

Indeed, Dr. Cowden has found that EFT is most effective whenever his clients are able to speak affirming statements that most accurately refute the cause of the depression, while tapping on the correct acupressure, or meridian points.

EFT has been reported to be anecdotally successful for healing people of a wide variety of emotional disorders, including depression. A few formal studies also substantiate its benefits. For instance, in one study published in 2012 in *The Journal of Nervous and Mental Disease,* nearly half of the people treated with EFT had less depression, as well as lowered levels of cortisol, a stress hormone that can cause harm to the body when levels are too high.

One of the benefits of EFT is that the basic techniques are simple to learn, and by studying the full procedure, which is outlined on the official EFT website: *EmoFree.com,* you may be able to resolve the underlying issues that are causing your depression without spending any money, and without having to leave your home. Furthermore, EFT is a safe therapy that doesn't harm your body in any way.

That said, if your depression is caused by deep-seated trauma, you might want to enlist the help of a healthcare practitioner trained in EFT, who can provide you with assistance using the techniques. You can find an EFT practitioner in your area by doing a search on the Association for Comprehensive Energy Psychology website: EnergyPsych.site-ym.com/search.

Alternatively, you could take the time to learn on your own the advanced techniques of EFT, which are available via the EFT site, but doing this may require more motivation, effort or time than the average depressed person has. EFT can be a useful healing tool, when other types of therapies, such as antidepressants, nutritional supplements or counseling, have proven to be inadequate.

CHAPTER THIRTY

REMAP Therapy

Reed Eye Movement Acupressure Psychotherapy (REMAP) is a unique energy psychology therapy invented by psychotherapist Steve B. Reed, which builds upon and combines principles of acupressure, mindfulness, breath regulation, eye movements and behavioral therapy. According to the REMAP Institute website, "REMAP is the innovative synthesis of mind-body therapy, brain science, powerful behavioral desensitization, counter-conditioning, mindfulness and simple, yet effective cognitive interventions. The total treatment effect is greater than the sum of the parts."

REMAP is comprised of three separate treatment methods: the full REMAP process, Quick REMAP and the REMAP Visual Field Treatment.

In REMAP, Steve Reed has completely reinvented the use of acupressure for the purpose of easing emotional distress. Dr. Cowden has found REMAP to be far more effective and to produce faster results than EFT (Emotional Freedom Techniques), EMDR (Eye Movement Desensitization and Reprocessing) or other mind-body therapies alone.

According to Dr. Cowden, Reed found that tapping on acupuncture meridians while repeating affirmations, as is done in EFT, was not always sufficient to heal his clients of post-traumatic stress disorder (PTSD), anxiety and depression caused by severe trauma. So he invented REMAP, which utilizes several effective psychotherapeutic interventions in combination with his original discoveries about bioenergetic medicine. He found that in some cases, this method would often resolve his clients' post-traumatic stress disorder after just a session or two of therapy.

REMAP functions by helping to retrain your limbic system, which is a complex system of nerves and networks that encompasses many parts of your brain, such as the hypothalamus, hippocampus and amygdala. These parts of your brain are all concerned with the primitive "fight-or-flight" reflex, instinct and emotions. Your limbic system also influences your autonomic nervous system, which then influences your neuroendocrine system, or your hormones and neurotransmitters, and consequently, your mood!

REMAP retrains and calms your limbic system, or midbrain, so that it no longer associates past traumatic events with pain, and no longer responds with a conditioned "fight-or-flight" response to current events. In this manner, it desensitizes you to specific past events that still cause emotional distress and can help you to resolve symptoms of anxiety, panic, stress and depression that are associated with past trauma.

For the full REMAP process, practitioners help you to identify specific painful events that continue to cause you emotional distress or to over-react. Next, they help you to connect with the physical sensations and emotions that are related to those events.

They then show you how to activate different points along a single acupuncture meridian of your body, by applying gentle pressure to the specific acupoints (rather than tapping only on the meridian terminal points, as in EFT). The meridian that you treat is the one that has been found through REMAP's diagnostic process to be the pathway in need of the greatest treatment.

REMAP calms the emotional midbrain, soothes the sympathetic nervous system and enables you to become desensitized to the pain that was linked to the distressing memory.

So, for instance, if you have fear as a predominant emotion, your practitioner might have you apply acupressure to different points all along your kidney meridian (in traditional Chinese medicine, fear is often associated with the kidneys), starting at one end of the kidney meridian and ending at the other end of the meridian.

Quick REMAP works in much the same way (as the full REMAP process), but instead of treating an entire meridian, it utilizes several key acupoints. The usefulness of these acupoints for healing the body has been proven at the Harvard and Yale Schools of Medicine. They are also known and regarded in Traditional Chinese medicine as highly potent acupressure points that can heal the body from a variety of conditions.

Dr. Cowden has found the Alpha-Stim®, light and sound machine, EFT, REMAP and Biomat therapies to all be particularly helpful for reducing acute anxiety, and the Clear Mind neurofeedback device and EMDR (Chapter 31) to be helpful for reducing chronic, long-term anxiety.

REMAP is primarily oriented toward treating the emotional midbrain. However, occasionally the thinking brain (cortex) can become involved in triggering distress by creating vivid stories and mental movies that are upsetting. For such situations, REMAP will utilize a three-part cognitive intervention in which you speak affirmations of objective truth, to counter the negative thoughts that are automatically triggered by your limbic system. This will stop the cortex from triggering false alarm reflexes in the limbic system.

While the REMAP treatment methods may be sufficient for helping you to find relief from your emotional distress, it can be useful at times to have a REMAP practitioner that is also trained in EMDR follow up a REMAP session with an EMDR treatment. This can enable you to further process the cognitive aspect of the emotional problem.

One of the benefits of both the full REMAP process and Quick REMAP is that you can often experience positive results much more quickly than with conventional psychotherapy or other mind-body tapping/affirmation-oriented therapies. Also, it doesn't require you to dig deep into past memories, which can be traumatizing for some people if they are not handled properly.

REMAP incorporates some eye movement elements into the technique but these movements are completely different from those that are used in EMDR. The REMAP eye circle technique, for instance, allows you to more accurately access a memory in preparation for utilizing a variety of strategies to soothe the midbrain's "fight-or-flight" response.

The REMAP interventions are able to anesthetize the intense emotions behind an upsetting memory. So, just as you would be given an anesthetic before undergoing a painful surgery, so REMAP provides an anesthesia of sorts while you undergo the process of emotional healing.

For more information on REMAP and where you can find a certified REMAP practitioner, we encourage you to visit the REMAP Institute website: *RemapInstitute.org*. You can also get further information about REMAP at *Remap.net*

I have seen many patients obtain radical benefits from REMAP therapy. For example, a healthcare practitioner once came to me with suicidal depression and panic. She was very anxious and couldn't sleep. She had made a bad investment decision that she believed would cause her to lose her home and practice. The situation caused her to be so upset that she couldn't sleep and was very depressed. She came to my office because she didn't want to go to a hospital where she would be reported to her licensing board and have to risk losing her license to practice. I did REMAP tapping on her, followed by EMDR. I also gave her two energetically-imprinted drainage remedies and two other energetically-imprinted herbal remedies to help release the emotions. As a result of doing those few things, she went from being suicidal and depressed and severely anxious, to having almost no depression or anxiety, in less than two hours.   —Dr. Lee Cowden

CHAPTER THIRTY-ONE

EMDR

EMDR (Eye Movement Desensitization and Reprocessing) is a well-established healing modality that utilizes principles of psychotherapy, along with one of several types of sensory input, such as side-to-side eye movements, hand-tapping, or audio stimulation, to process traumatic or disturbing memories that can lead to a wide range of problems including mood disorders such as depression.

According to therapist and physician Karl Lehman, MD, in his article, "Theophostic & EMDR: F.A.Q.'s and Common Misunderstandings", "EMDR has the strongest empirical research support of any treatment modality for the healing of psychological trauma."

You can usually obtain more positive results with EMDR therapy more quickly than with conventional psychotherapy or counseling. One to four sessions of EMDR can often bring about as much trauma resolution as a year of conventional psychotherapy.

The developer of EMDR, Dr. Francine Shapiro, PhD,

> EMDR therapy helps you to access and process memories
> that are negatively affecting you, in order to bring them to an
> adaptive resolution. You do side-to-side eye movements, or
> listen to audio sounds, which serve to help your brain to make
> needed associations and "digest" the memories, even those
> that you only vaguely remember or may have completely
> forgotten.

> At the same time, the mental health professional guides
> your focus of attention to ensure that the memory is fully
> processed, which then changes your negative emotions into
> positive ones, creates a new (more positive) perspective, and
> transforms the traumatic memory into a source of resilience.

> The new associations created by the processing can eliminate
> your emotional distress and depression caused by these past
> memories, while encouraging you to develop new, more
> beneficial beliefs and thought patterns.

EMDR was originally developed to treat adults who were
suffering from post-traumatic stress disorder; however, it can
also be used to treat depression associated with any type of
negative past experience.

You can usually obtain more positive results with EMDR
therapy more quickly than with conventional psychotherapy
or counseling. One to four sessions of EMDR can often bring
about as much trauma resolution as a year of conventional
psychotherapy.

According to the EMDR Institute, Inc.,

… studies show that the mind can heal from psychological trauma much as the body recovers from physical trauma. When you cut your hand, your body works to close the wound. If a foreign object or repeated injury irritates the wound, it festers and causes pain. Once the block is removed, healing resumes.

EMDR therapy demonstrates that a similar sequence of events occurs with mental processes. The brain's information processing system naturally moves toward mental health. If the system is blocked or imbalanced by the impact of a disturbing event, the emotional wound festers and can cause intense suffering. Once the block is removed, healing resumes. Using the detailed protocols and procedures learned in EMDR training sessions, clinicians help clients activate their natural healing processes.

The effectiveness of EMDR is backed by substantial research and clinical studies. According to therapist and physician Karl Lehman, MD, in his article, "Theophostic & EMDR: F.A.Q.'s and Common Misunderstandings,"

EMDR has the strongest empirical research support of any treatment modality for the healing of psychological trauma. SPECT scan research documents brain activity changes with EMDR. A number of controlled studies indicate that EMDR is a valid treatment for civilian PTSD. A meta-analysis looking at 59 studies of PTSD treatments indicated that EMDR is effective for reducing symptoms of PTSD.

Other controlled studies have shown EMDR to be effective for treating phobias, stress in law enforcement employees, and distress experienced by traumatized children. My summary assessment of research finding positive results is that studies done by mental health professionals who actually use EMDR in their own professional work consistently show dramatic benefit.

> **Homeopathy is a type of bioenergetic medicine that was invented in 1796 by the German physician Samuel Hahnemann. It is based on the idea of like cures like; meaning, a substance that causes symptoms of disease in a healthy person will cure those same symptoms in a person who is sick.**

One disadvantage of EMDR over other types of therapies is that it requires you to access potentially traumatic memories, which may be difficult and undesirable if the memories are very disturbing. If your practitioner isn't properly trained, you can become re-traumatized, especially if you aren't ready to revisit those memories.

Also, EMDR is unlikely to heal you from depression if the depression isn't caused by past trauma. If your depression is caused by environmental toxicity, for example, or an infection, or a nutritional deficiency, then EMDR may not resolve it. It is, however, a worthwhile therapy to consider if you have a strong history of trauma that you believe is linked to your current feelings.

To find a practitioner in your area that does EMDR, visit the EMDR International Association: *Emdria.org/* and click on the link, Find a Therapist.

Bioenergetic Treatments for Anxiety

Many of us today are anxious. And like depression, anxiety is caused by a variety of factors, including past traumas in our lives, current stressors, a poor diet and illness, among other things.

Many of today's chronic health conditions, including some types of anxiety, are caused by environmental toxins. If you suspect toxicity to be a main cause of your anxiety, homotoxicology remedies that support your detoxification organs can not only help you to detoxify, but also relieve the symptoms of anxiety.

Anxiety, like depression, is a condition that affects not only your emotions, but also your mind and body. If you are anxious, you might experience a constant but vague sense of nervousness or unease, or you might have intense feelings of fear, panic and dread, among other uncomfortable emotions. If you suffer from anxiety, you'll tend to be a worrier. The worries will often have to do with real or perceived threats to your own safety and well-being, or that of the people that you love.

If you suffer from anxiety, you may also have physical symptoms such as heart palpitations, dizziness, light-headedness, muscle tightness, shortness of breath, and digestive or nervous system problems—even pain. Insomnia is also common.

All of the treatments that we described in the previous sections on *Bioenergetic Treatments for Insomnia and Depression* are also useful for treating anxiety, especially when the anxiety is related to past traumatic events.

Dr. Cowden has found the Alpha-Stim®, light and sound machine, EFT, REMAP and Biomat therapies to all be particularly helpful for reducing acute anxiety, and the Clear Mind neurofeedback device and EMDR to be helpful for reducing chronic, long-term anxiety.

In the following chapters, we describe some additional treatments for anxiety, which are inexpensive, effective and powerful for alleviating symptoms of both acute and long-term anxiety. These include Bach and other flower remedies, and energetically imprinted herbal remedies. Similarly, these treatments can also be helpful for relieving symptoms of depression, so there is considerable overlap in usefulness among the many therapies and remedies that we describe in this book.

CHAPTER THIRTY-TWO

Homeopathy, Homotoxicology and Energetically Imprinted Remedies

Homeopathic and other energy remedies are great to use if you are sensitive to other therapies, don't have the time or money to visit a therapist, or don't want to do manual techniques that require time and effort, such as EFT. The remedies are generally inexpensive and gentle and require less of an investment of time and energy than the other healing modalities that we describe in this book.

Bioenergetic tools for healing aren't limited to electromagnetic devices or manual therapies. They also include oral homeopathic and energetically-imprinted remedies that contain either the energetic imprint of a physical substance, such as an herb or toxin; the energy of an infectious microbe (which is used to treat disease in a vaccine-like manner), or the energetic signature or imprint of some other substance, which is used either to potentiate the effects of another substance or create a healing response in the body.

The NutraMedix product Amantilla is one example of an energetically- imprinted valerian root remedy that we have found to be very valuable for calming the body and mind and reducing symptoms of acute anxiety.

These energetic remedies can be used to treat anything from minor ailments to severe disease. For the purposes of this book, we will only be describing their usefulness for treating anxiety. In the following sections, we provide some basic information about homeopathy and energetically imprinted herbal and flower remedies, all of which are useful for reducing or eliminating symptoms of anxiety, especially acute anxiety, or anxiety caused by current stressors in your life.

Homeopathic and other energy remedies are great to use if you are sensitive to other therapies, don't have the time or money to visit a therapist, or don't want to do manual techniques that require time and effort, such as EFT. The remedies are generally inexpensive and gentle and require less of an investment of time and energy than the other healing modalities that we describe in this book.

In order to obtain the most benefit from them, however, it's best to work with a holistic healthcare practitioner, ideally, a homeopath or other doctor experienced in their use and who thoroughly understands how to select an appropriate remedy based on the root cause of your anxiety.

You may need multiple remedies, depending upon whether your anxiety is due to past trauma, acute situational stress, or a biochemical imbalance resulting from disease or a nutritional deficiency. Some remedies are more powerful than others, and will vary in their effectiveness, depending on the root cause of your anxiety and the skill of the practitioner who is helping you.

We also describe some remedies that you can purchase over-the-counter and try out on your own. You may find that these self-prescribed remedies are sufficient to relieve your anxiety, in which case you would not need to visit a health care practitioner.

Dr. Edward Bach (1886–1936), a British physician and homeopath, developed the Bach flower remedies after he discovered that the energies of different flowers worked to resolve troubling emotions, and that each flower was useful for healing a different emotional condition.

Many energetic remedies are founded upon principles of homeopathy, which is a type of bioenergetic medicine that was invented in 1796 by the German physician Samuel Hahnemann. It is based on the idea of like cures like; meaning, a substance that causes symptoms of disease in a healthy person will cure those same symptoms in a person who is sick, when the correct dilution is given. In this regard, it functions somewhat like a vaccine or a series of allergy injections.

Homeopathic remedies, which are usually the energetic blueprint of different biochemical substances, microbes or disease-causing agents, are prescribed according to your constitution, symptoms, personal characteristics and history. Some practitioners use electrodermal screening or muscle testing to guide their recommendations for a homeopathic remedy.

Homotoxicology is a branch of homeopathy developed by Dr. Hans Henrich Reckeweg (Germany) in the early 1900s that is based on the principles of classical homeopathy, but practitioners that utilize it place more emphasis on the physical manifestations of disease, rather than your constitution and history, when determining what remedies to prescribe. Prescriptions are also based upon your symptoms and clinical findings, as is done in conventional medicine, as well as the current stressors in your life.

Classical homeopathic remedy prescriptions are often based upon a single substance, whereas in homotoxicology, multiple remedies are often combined in such a way to address the greatest amount of toxic and functional problems in your body. The objective in homotoxicology is to reduce the effects of stress and toxins upon your body, while classical homeopathy aims to resolve the root cause of your disease. As such, classical homeopathy is designed to create a healing response that radically moves your entire body towards wellness. Both classical homeopathy and homotoxicology can resolve symptoms by balancing your body's energy, but through different means.

Classical homeopathic remedies, when properly prescribed, can be much more powerful and produce more dramatic results in the short term than homotoxicology remedies, since classical homeopathy addresses the root cause of anxiety, rather than just its symptoms. A single remedy taken for a week can completely reverse a severe anxiety disorder, if the remedy gets to the root cause, while the effects of homotoxicology remedies seem to be more cumulative.

Many of today's chronic health conditions, including some types of anxiety, are caused by environmental toxins, so if you suspect toxicity to be a main cause of your anxiety, homotoxicology remedies that support your detoxification organs—the kidneys, liver and lymphatic system, for instance—can not only help you to detoxify, but also relieve the symptoms of anxiety. Pekana (*Pekana.com*), Heel (*Heel.com*) and NutraMedix (*NutraMedix.com*) are a few companies that make exceptional homotoxicology-type remedies for organ support.

Otherwise, if you have long-term chronic anxiety, or acute anxiety caused by other factors besides toxins, we recommend consulting with a classical homeopath that can help to prescribe the best remedy for your needs. You can find a local homeopath in your area by consulting the National Center for Homeopathy: HomeopathyCenter.org or The Homeopathic Academy of Naturopathic Physicians: *HANP.net*. Popular websites such as homeopathic-md-do.com and homeopathy-cures.com also have homeopathic practitioner lists.

ENERGETICALLY IMPRINTED HERBAL REMEDIES

Energetically imprinted remedies are similar to homeopathic remedies in that they can sometimes contain the energetic signature of one or more physical substances. Unlike homeopathy, however, they don't aim to cure via the principle of "like cures like." Instead, they shift your energy to create a specific healing response in an organ or set of tissues.

So, for instance, herbal remedies can be energetically imprinted with frequencies that potentiate the effects of the herbs upon your body. Valerian root, for example, alleviates anxiety by relaxing your nervous system. However, when you imprint it with specific energetic frequencies, then it becomes even more effective because the frequencies cause it to act upon more energetic cellular receptors in your body. The herbal component of the remedy will act upon some of your nervous system receptors, while the imprinted energies will act upon additional energetic cellular receptors, thereby potentiating the effects of the herb.

> If unconscious emotional conflicts remain unresolved in your body, it leads to a reduced flow of energy throughout the body which then sets the stage for a variety of physical, mental and/or emotional disorders to occur.

The NutraMedix product Amantilla is one example of an energetically-imprinted valerian root remedy that we have found to be very valuable for calming the body and mind and reducing symptoms of acute anxiety. It combines valerian root with the energetic frequencies of other flowers, neurotransmitters and other substances.

The valerian root in Amantilla has an effect upon certain chemical receptors on the cell's surface, while the energetic signal of passionflower and other substances imprinted into the remedy have a different effect. So who knows if you are getting more effect from the herb that is the carrier for the energies, or the quantum energies themselves! In any case, both function to relax your nervous system and relieve symptoms of anxiety.

CHAPTER THIRTY-THREE

Bach Flower Remedies

Bach flower remedies are another type of homeopathic remedy that may be especially useful for alleviating symptoms of anxiety. Unlike pharmaceutical medications, which only target your symptoms, Bach Flower remedies can be prescribed according to the type of anxiety that you suffer from.

> To find a Bach flower practitioner, visit the Bach Centre website, which contains a worldwide guide of practitioners that do Bach Flower Therapy: *BachCentre.com.*

Dr. Edward Bach (1886–1936), a British physician and homeopath, developed the Bach flower remedies after he discovered that the energies of different flowers worked to resolve troubling emotions, and that each flower was useful for healing a different emotional condition.

Dr. Bach first captured the energy of flowers by dripping water over their surface and then catching that water in a glass. Today, Bach remedies are made by boiling the flowers to extract their essence. They contain no chemicals whatsoever—only the energy of the flower.

Some benefits of the Bach Flower remedies are that they are safe to use and inexpensive, and you can take them without the guidance of a healthcare practitioner. So even if you make a mistake and choose a remedy that's less than optimal for you, it won't harm you. We recommend purchasing a guide on the remedies, or doing an Internet search on the common uses of different flowers, and then trying some remedies on your own.

That said, as with the other therapies mentioned in this book, you might see faster or better results if you work with a certified Bach Flower Practitioner, who can prepare special Bach Flower Remedy formulations according to your specific needs. This might be especially important if you suffer from deep-seated or severe anxiety issues.

Below are some common Bach Flower Remedies and the types of anxiety conditions that they are commonly used to treat, according to The Bach Centre (*BachCentre.com*), and The Original Bach Flower Remedies website (*bachflower.com*). We also recommend consulting Dr. Bach's book, *The Bach Flower Remedies*, for more information on these and other remedies.

Red Chestnut This is a good choice of remedy if you worry excessively about the well-being of your children or other close family members.

Mimulus According to Dr. Bach, this remedy is good for treating "Fear of worldly things, illness, pain, accidents, poverty, of dark, of being alone, of misfortune. The fears of everyday life. These people quietly and secretly bear their dread; they do not freely speak of it to others." It is also useful for treating phobias, such as the fear of flying, small spaces, public speaking, etc.

Aspen This is useful if you have vague symptoms of anxiety that you can't trace to a particular cause, or terror that something awful is going to happen, even though you don't know what.

Rock Rose This remedy is beneficial if you suffer from panic attacks, or are extremely terrified or frightened about something.

Crab Apple This is useful if your anxiety is related to feeling unclean or unacceptable in some way. It is also useful if you have anxiety about contamination, dirt or germs.

Cherry Plum This is useful for quelling fears of losing your mind, or losing control.

Larch According to Dr. Bach, this remedy is good "For those who do not consider themselves as good or capable as those around them, who expect failure, who feel that they will never be a success, and so do not venture or make a strong enough attempt to succeed."

Centaury This remedy is a good choice if you have fears of standing up for yourself.

Cerato This remedy is useful for alleviating fears about making the wrong decisions.

Star of Bethlehem This remedy is used if you have anxiety caused by a traumatic event or shock.

You can take multiple Bach Flower remedies simultaneously, but most Bach Flower remedy practitioners will only prescribe one to four remedies at a time to their clients, even though they might feel like they could benefit from all 38 Flower Essences!

One well-known Bach remedy that is commonly sold in health food stores, called the Bach Rescue Remedy, is comprised of five remedies. This product is useful if you have recently suffered from anxiety related to a shock or trauma.

If you aren't sure which remedies would best suit you, a Bach flower practitioner can help you to formulate a protocol. If your anxiety is deeply rooted, long-standing or severe, consider consulting with a practitioner and doing additional strategies for anxiety, such as psychotherapy or EMDR.

The Bach flower remedies were among the first flower remedies developed to treat emotional conditions, but there are many other types of flower remedies that you may find to be helpful for treating your anxiety if one or more of the Bach flower remedies don't work.

These include Bush flower remedies from Australia, North American and South American flower remedies. For more information on these and other types of flowers, we recommend checking out the Flower Essence Society (FES) website: *flowersociety.org/*. This is an international membership organization of health practitioners, researchers and others dedicated to increasing the knowledge of flower essence therapy.

To find a Bach flower practitioner, visit the Bach Centre website, which contains a worldwide guide of practitioners that do Bach Flower Therapy: *bachcentre.com.*

CHAPTER THIRTY-FOUR

Other Bioenergetic Therapies for Anxiety

The energy circulation pathway of the index finger in Oriental medicine is associated with fear, and that of your middle finger with unresolved anger, so holding your left middle finger while forgiving those people with whom you are angry, can help to resolve any anger that you might have while helping you to relax.

RUBIMED THERAPY

Rubimed™ is a healing modality from Europe that has now also been used in North America for over a decade. According to the Rubimed website: www.Rubimed.com, Rubimed was developed by Dr. Reimar Banis, a German physician and researcher, and is based upon principles found in biophysics, homeopathy and psychology, and the idea that "a harmonious and free-flowing energy system is important for mental, emotional and physical health."

Rubimed practitioners utilize complex homeopathic-like remedies to remove the programming and energetic influence of emotional conflicts that cause disease.

According to the Rubimed website, psychomatic energetics, one of the main principles upon which Rubimed is based, illness is associated with emotional trauma, which becomes repressed into the subconscious and is stored in the body's energy field. If unconscious emotional conflicts remain unresolved in your body, it leads to a reduced flow of energy throughout your body which then sets the stage for a variety of physical, mental and/or emotional disorders to occur.

Rubimed practitioners utilize complex homeopathic-like remedies to remove the programming and energetic influence of emotional conflicts that cause disease. The remedies that you need are determined based on the results of energetic testing—either electrodermal screening or muscle testing.

Rubimed™ remedies have been anecdotally and clinically proven to resolve chronic illness and health problems caused by psychological trauma, anxiety and stress. For more information about this therapy and to find a practitioner in your state or country that does Rubimed, visit: *Rubimed.com*, or *Terra-Medica.com*

TKM

The King Method, which was described earlier in this book, has a simple technique that you can do to reduce acute symptoms of stress and anxiety. While sitting in a lounger or lying down (or at least sitting in a very comfortable chair) with no jewelry, metal belt buckles or wire-rimmed glasses on, breathe continuously and deeply in through your nose and out through your nose or mouth while touching your tongue to the roof of your mouth.

As you continue to breathe this way, hold your middle and index fingers of your left hand together with your right hand. As you do this, forgive everyone with whom you are angry as you visualize their faces, one at a time with your eyes closed.

The energy circulation pathway of the index finger in Oriental medicine is associated with fear, and that of your middle finger with unresolved anger, so holding your left middle finger while forgiving those with whom you are angry, can help to resolve that anger more easily and help you to relax.

Then, grasp your left thumb and index finger together simultaneously. The energy circulation pathway of the index finger, as we previously mentioned, is associated with fear, while the thumb is associated with worry. As you do this technique, you can ask God to help you to release all feelings of fear and worry and/or you can visualize yourself releasing more fear and worry every time you breathe out.

Holding these fingers while praying or speaking affirmations can help you to quell unhealthy emotions or thoughts that lead to anxiety.

A similar technique works for resolving other emotions. For instance, if you are suffering from sadness and grief, grasp your ring finger, which is the finger associated with grief in Chinese medicine. As you do this, pray and ask God to take away the sadness and grief that you are feeling and/or visualize yourself releasing sadness and grief with each exhaled breath.

If you are struggling with feelings of inadequacy, spend a few minutes holding your little finger, while asking God to help you to see yourself as adequate and acceptable and/or visualizing each inhaled breath bringing into you more self-worth, and seeing each exhaled breath release all feelings of inadequacy.

As you do this therapy, hold each digit for four to five minutes as you pray or recite affirmations that are appropriate to that digit's corresponding emotion, which will then help you to release that emotion. Since worry is associated with the thumb, and fear is associated with the index finger, if you hold these two fingers together at the same time, you will be dealing with both of these emotions simultaneously.

Sometime during this process you may fall asleep, especially if you don't dwell on the negative things that happened that day or worry about what might happen the next day.

Some people who have done this technique have also found that their mind and body can relax to a greater extent if, during this technique, they also visualize themselves in an enjoyable vacation spot, and remember that place vividly with all of their senses—sight, sound, taste, touch and smell—as they breathe in and out deeply, and hold their left index finger and left thumb with their right hand. Remembering such a place with all of your senses can crowd out of your mind the thoughts that were causing the emotional distress.

This relaxation technique represents a very simple application of TKM for depression and anxiety. More complex sequences are used to treat other conditions.

For a simplified version of the above TKM sequence, grasp your left index finger and thumb with your right hand. Energy pathways for your nervous system and your body's neurotransmitters are found on the index finger, and a lymphatic system pathway is found on the thumb. Nervous people tend to have a clogged lymphatic system and overly active nervous system, so if you hold your left index and thumb together with your right hand for four to five minutes, then this will help to dissipate the excess energy in these energy pathways, and redistribute it into other energy pathways on the palm surface of your right hand. If you breathe deeply and visualize yourself in a relaxing place while you do this, it will increase the effectiveness of this technique.

In Summary

By now we hope that we've convinced you that bioenergetic medicine offers some fantastic therapies for maintaining wellness, as well as for healing your body from a variety of conditions, including those that we describe in this book. If used appropriately, these modalities are generally safer, gentler, faster acting, and more effective than pharmaceutical drugs or surgical treatments. They can also help to heal you when other types of holistic treatments may have failed to do so.

We hope that this book has helped you to believe that your symptoms can be effectively diagnosed and overcome, and that you can feel better than you ever have before, no matter how many doctors you may have seen, or how many other therapies you have tried. Take heart—if conventional or chemical medicine hasn't provided you with the answers that you need, chances are, bioenergetic medicine can!

Finding the tools that will best suit you may be somewhat of a trial and error process. Still, we believe that the chances are good that you will eventually find at least a few strategies in this book that will help bring you to a higher level of well-being in your journey toward wellness, so that you can experience life more fully and abundantly.

Bioenergetic Medicine— for Detoxifying Your Body and Treating Scars

Scars block the flow of energy through acupuncture meridians. To restore proper energy flow through these meridians, simply run a laser pointer over your scar for a few minutes daily for several weeks.

LASER ENERGETIC DETOXIFICATION (LED)

I have developed an innovative strategy for removing environmental toxins from the body, called Laser Energetic Detoxification. This strategy combines homeopathy with light therapy, and is a rapid, gentle, and non-invasive method for removing chemicals, heavy metals, sulfa drug residue and food/chemical sensitivities from the body. —Dr. Lee Cowden

For LED, a practitioner uses a special technology to imprint the energetic frequencies of different toxic chemical substances and allergenic foods into a clear-glass vial containing a liquid remedy of some type.

He or she then uses an infrared light and a laser to pass light through the vial, sweeping that light over the patient's body in a specific fashion. The light effectively transfers the energetic information from the vial into the body and stimulates the body to remove whatever toxins are contained within the vial. It also diminishes the patient's, or client's, allergic reactions to whatever allergens are in the vial.

LED is based upon homeopathy, quantum physics, and detoxification principles. Usually, homeopathic remedies are taken under the tongue as pellets or liquid drops. However, for LED, light is used to deliver the homeopathic remedy into the body.

Before doing an LED session, practitioners assess their patients for chemical toxins through muscle testing or via an electrodermal screening system such as the ZYTO. These tests can reveal whether sulfur-based compounds, chemical toxins, heavy metals, pharmaceuticals and other toxins are adversely affecting them.

One LED session can often remove more toxins from your body than several months of oral detoxification therapy, and when done periodically, patients recover from chronic conditions much more quickly. For more information about LED, we encourage you to visit the Academy of Comprehensive Integrative Medicine website: *AcimConnect.com.*

To date, only a few health care practitioners do LED. A list of practitioners that do LED can be found at The Academy for Comprehensive Integrative Medicine website: *AcimConnect.com*.

> I once had a patient who rarely slept more than two hours at a time, and no more than four hours per night. She had tried all kinds of natural therapies, herbs, and other treatments. Energetic testing results suggested that she had an energetic autoimmunity to her own neurotransmitters, because of pesticides that were in her brain.
>
> So I created a homeopathic homaccord remedy containing these pesticides then shone a laser light through the vial that contained the pesticides, onto her body. The first night after her treatment, she slept 10 hours, and then 8 hours the following night! Since that one LED treatment, she has continued to sleep 7-8 hours per night. —Dr. Lee Cowden

CLAY THERAPY

Anything that disrupts your body's energy flow through its acupuncture meridians will have a negative effect upon it. Scars, for instance, block the flow of energy through acupuncture meridians. To restore proper energy flow through these meridians, simply run a laser pointer over your scar for a few minutes daily for several

To do clay mud treatments, mix enough pure water with bentonite clay powder to make a mud, and then "paint" that mixture over your scar areas. Leave it there for approximately ten minutes, and then rinse it off.

weeks. Alternatively, you can do clay mud treatments, which will pull toxins from your scars and restore proper energy flow to your body.

To do clay mud treatments, mix enough pure water with bentonite clay powder to make a mud, and then "paint" that mixture over your scar areas. Leave it there for approximately ten minutes, and then rinse it off. Repeat the procedure at least two more times that same day.

It's most essential for women who have had babies by vaginal delivery to treat any scar tissue resulting from a vaginal tear or from an episiotomy, which is a common surgical procedure done at childbirth in order to prevent vaginal tears. Men who have been circumcised should also treat the area of circumcision, since this procedure also blocks energy flow through the meridians.

Some particularly excellent detoxification products from NutraMedix include: Burbur Detox, Parsley Detox, Pinella Brain and Nerve Cleanse, Sparga, Zeolite and Zeolite-HP. You can find these at: NutraMedix.com.

It's not usually a good idea to treat all of the scars on your body at once, because scar treatment can cause your body to mobilize many toxins, which can overload the detoxification organs and cause detoxification symptoms. For this reason, we recommend treating only four to five inches of scar tissue daily. Treating your scars can help to re-establish proper energy flow throughout your body, which in turn will help you to improve your overall health.

REFLEXOLOGY

Reflexology, which we briefly described earlier in this book, is a form of bodywork that focuses primarily on the soles of the feet and the palms of the hands. According to the principles of reflexology, when you apply pressure to specific areas of your palms and soles, it also affects the organs, glands, and other parts of your body that are linked via the meridian system to that area of your foot or hand.

Every tender spot on your hands or feet corresponds to a physical distress somewhere in your body. You can find out which of your organs is being distressed by looking up a reflexology chart on the Internet and seeing which organ or body part on the chart corresponds to the point or points on your palms and soles that are tender.

Doing reflexology is easy. After you find the tender nodules or spots on your palms or the soles of your feet, press on those areas, and massage them in a clockwise fashion until you feel no more discomfort.

If you have a chronic illness, learning reflexology is worthwhile because doing this simple technique can help to strengthen your organs, eliminate toxins, increase your energy, reduce pain, alleviate cognitive symptoms and sometimes even reduce insomnia, depression and anxiety.

For more information on reflexology, visit: *Reflexology-usa.net.*

ISONOSODES

Isonosodes are homeopathic remedies that you can make on your own, and which are prepared from microbial secretions that come from your own body and are useful for detoxifying it from environmental toxins and microbes. You can make isonosodes from your own urine, for instance. Urine is great to use because it is known to contain fragments of antibodies that function like a vaccine when they are delivered back to your body.

Auto-urine therapy dates back to ancient cultures. Egyptian, Chinese and Indian documents and medical texts all mention the benefits of urine as a remedy.

Contrary to what most of us probably think, urine isn't a byproduct of your body's waste removal system but of its blood filtration system. Nutrient-filled blood passes first through your liver. The liver removes many toxins from the blood and excretes them as solid waste. The purified blood is then filtered again through the kidneys, and anything that remains in the blood that your body doesn't need is collected in a sterile, watery solution that is the urine.

One LED session can often remove more toxins from your body than several months of oral detoxification therapy, and when done periodically, patients recover from chronic conditions much more quickly.

To make an isonosode from urine, simply take an empty dropper bottle, and pour a bit of your first morning urine into that bottle, so that it fills up about 10 percent of the bottle. Then, fill the bottle to the shoulder with purified, spring or distilled water. Then, succuss, (shake it forcefully) 50 to 100 times. Pour out 9/10 of the solution and fill the bottle to the shoulder again with water.

Succuss the bottle a second time, and again, pour out 9/10 of the solution, as before. Then, fill the bottle to the shoulder with Polish potato vodka or organic grape wine alcohol. Cap the bottle and succuss it a third time. By diluting and succussing the solution three times, it creates what is called a 3X homeopathic remedy.

Take five to ten drops of this solution twice daily for several weeks. Smaller people should take a dosage of about five drops; larger people should take ten. This will help you to remove a variety of toxins and infectious microbes from your body.

Homeopathic Drainage Remedies

Homeopathic drainage or homotoxicology remedies also help to support your body's natural detoxification processes. They are especially important to use during the initial phases of detoxification, when you are trying to eliminate lots of contaminants from your body, or when you are sick and have compromised organ function.

These remedies strengthen your detoxification organs—particularly the liver, kidneys and lymphatic system—and cause them to be more efficient and effective at removing toxins.

As we mentioned earlier in this book, Pekana and Heel make excellent homotoxicology remedies, and NutraMedix makes herbal products that have homeopathic-like effects upon the body. Some particularly excellent detoxification products from NutraMedix include: Burbur Detox, Parsley Detox, Pinella Brain and Nerve Cleanse, Sparga, Zeolite and Zeolite-HP. You can find these at: *NutraMedix.com.*

Further Reading and References

CHAPTERS 3-5

Proof We Are Energetic Beings/ Why Bioenergetic Medicine?/ Where Our Energy Comes From and How We Use It

Gallo, F. "Articles Evidencing the Existence of Energy Meridians." EF-TUniverse.com. Retrieved on April 14, 2014 from: *eftuniverse.com/index.php?option=com_content&view=article&id=2479*

Gordon, D. MRI (28 Dec. 1998) Evidence of Acupuncture. *The Orange County Register*. Retrieved on April 14, 2014 from: *Acupuncture Doc. com. http://www.acupuncturedoc.com/scientif.htm*

Membrane Potential. Wikipedia. Retrieved on April 14, 2014 from: *wikipedia.org/wiki/Membrane_potential*

Voll, R. *Biontology.com*. Retrieved on April 14, 2014 from: *biontology.com/wp-content/uploads/2012/08/Voll.pdf*

CHAPTERS 5-6

EMR Pollution/Geopathic Stress

Carpenter, D.O. "Human disease resulting from exposure to electromagnetic fields." *Rev Environ Health.* (2013);28(4):159-72. doi: 10.1515/reveh-2013-0016

Carlo, G. (2007). "The Hidden Dangers of Cell Phone Radiation." *Life Extension Magazine*. Retrieved on March 7, 2012 from: *lef.org/magazine/mag2007/aug2007_report_cellphone_radiation_01.htm*

Cherry, Neil. (2002-2005). "Epidemiological Studies of Enhanced Brain/CNS Cancer Incidence and Mortality from EMR and EMF Exposures." Lincoln University, Canterbury, NZ.

Cherry, Neil. (2002-2005). "Evidence that EMF/EMR Causes Leukaemia/Lymphoma in Adults and Children." Lincoln University, Canterbury, NZ.

Dubrov, A. "Geopathic Zones and Oncological Diseases." Federal Scientific &-Clinical Experimental Center of Tradition Methods of Diagnostics and Medical Treatment of Roszdav RF Moscow, Russia. June 2008 seminar in Druskininkai, Lithuania

Earthing products: *earthinginstitute.net*

Electromagnetic Health (website of Camilla Rees, MBA): *electromagnetichealth.org*

Electrosensor and other EMF products: *lessemf.com/gauss.html*

EMF Safety Store: *emfsafetystore.com*

EMR Stop. (2010).Transcript Interview with Dr. Thomas M. Rau of the Para- celsus Clinic. Retrieved on Jan. 12, 2011 from: *emrstop.org/index. php?option=com_content&view=article&id=139:transcript-interview-with-dr- thomas-m-rau-of-the-swiss-paracelsus-clinic&catid=6:K.* (2010) *emrstop.org*

Fauteux, A. Electromagnetic Intolerance Elucidated. *EMFacts Consultancy*. Retrieved on Feb. 7, 2011 from: *emfacts.com/2012/01/electromagnetic-intolerance-elucidated/*

French Association for Research in Therapeutics against Cancer: *artac.info*

Geopathic Stress — superstition or fact. How does it affect our well-being? *Natural Science Medicine*. Retrieved on April 14, 2014 from: *naturalsciencemedicine.com/information/causes-of-illness/ geopathic-stress/*

Geopathic Stress and Cancer. *Healing Cancer Naturally*. Retrieved on April 14, 2014 from: *healingcancernaturally.com/geopathic-stress-and-cancer.html*

Hardell L1, Carlberg M, Söderqvist F, Mild KH. "Case-control study of the association between malignant brain tumours diagnosed between 2007 and 2009 and mobile and cordless phone use." *Int J Oncol.* (2013 Dec);43(6):1833-45. doi: 10.3892/ijo.2013.2111. Epub 2013 Sep 24

Memon products: *memonyourharmony.com*

Santini, R., Santini, P., Danze, J.M., Le Ruz, P., Seigne, M. "Symptoms experienced by people in vicinity of base stations: II. Incidences of age, duration of exposure, location of subjects in relation to the antennas and other electromagnetic factors." *Pathol. Biol.* (2003) 51:412-415.

Sirish, M. Why Cell Phone Towers Are So Bad for Your Health. *The Big Picture.* Retrieved on April 20, 2014 from: *drsirish.blogspot. com/2010/09/why-cell-phone-towers-are-so-bad-for.html.*

Stan Hartman, RadSafe, Boulder, Colorado: *radsafe.net*

Study Links Power Lines to Cancer. *British Medical Journal.* (2005) Retrieved on March 4, 2011 from: *powerlinefacts.com/large_study_links_ power_lines_to_leukemia.htm.*

The Institute of Building Biology + Ecology Neubeuern: *baubiolo- gie.de/ site/english.php*

The International Institute for Building Biology and Ecology: *hbelc.org/ findexpert/enviroconsult.html*

To do an antennae search: *antennasearch.com*

CHAPTERS 9-13

Do-It-Yourself and Doctors' Diagnostic Techniques

Muscle Testing, EDS, HRV, Chinese Pulse Testing and Thermography

Contact Regulation Thermography: *alfathermo.com* or *eidam.com.*

Dubowsky, J. Understanding Chinese Pulse Diagnosis. *Emperor's College of Traditional Oriental Medicine.* Retrieved on April 14, 2014 from: *emperors.edu/Qiblog/2012/08/pulse-power-understanding-tcm-pulse- diagnosis/*

Heart Rate Variability Testing- Heart Quest.com *hhrvhq.com*

ZYTO EDS devices: *ZYTO.com*

CHAPTERS 15-18

Bioenergetic Treatments for Fatigue – TKM, PEMF, Acupuncture, Earthing, EEG Biofeedback, etc.

BEMERAmerica.com

Dr. Oz on PEMF Therapy and Pain Relief *Dr. Magda Havas, PhD.* Retrieved on April 14, 2014 from: *magdahavas.com/category/ health-issues/pemf-therapy/*

Earthing Products: *EarthingInstitute.net*

Fishman, J. The history of acupuncture. *Acupuncture.com.acupuncture. com/education/theory/historyacu.htm*

Magnafield Device- MagnaCareUK. *magnacareuk.com/product/ magnafield/*

NutraMedix Adrenal Support. *nutramedix.com/store/pc/viewPrd. asp?idproduct=2&idcategory=3*

PEMF Devices: *PEMF.us* and *PEMF.com*

Studies: *pemf.com/en/studies.html*

PEMF-100: *PEMF.us, pemf.us/products.html*

PFG2Z. Pulsed Technologies: *pulsedtech.com/pfg2z.html*

Pulsed Electromagnetic Fields—How They Heal. *The Dr. Oz Show.* Retrieved on April 14, 2014 from: *doctoroz.com/videos/pulsed-electromagnetic-fields-how-they-heal*

Saunas: Momentum 98 Company, at: *momentum98.com*

TKM-The King Institute: *TheKingInstitute.org.*

CHAPTER 19-22

Bioenergetic Treatments for Pain- PEMF, TKM, LLLT, Acupuncture, Iontophoresis, Infrared Photonic Focal Detox, etc.

Acupuncture for Pain. *National Center for Complementary and Alternative Medicine. nccam.nih.gov/health/acupuncture/acupuncture-for-pain.htm*

BioActive Nutritionals Products: Viscum Force, Hepatotox, Lymph II and Nephroplex. *bioactivenutritional.com*

Bliss in a Bottle: *supergoodstuff.com*

Brosseau L1, Welch V, Wells G, Tugwell P, de Bie R, Gam A, Harman K, Shea B, Morin M. "Low level laser therapy for osteoarthritis and rheumatoid arthritis: a metaanalysis." *J Rheumatol.* 2000 Aug;27(8):1961-9.

Cheing GL1, Li X, Huang L, Kwan RL, Cheung KK. "Pulsed electromagnetic fields (PEMF) promote early wound healing and myofibroblast proliferation in diabetic rats." *Bioelectromagnetics* (2014 Apr);35(3):161-9. doi: 10.1002/bem.21832. Epub 2014 Jan 3.

Gross AR1, Dziengo S, Boers O, Goldsmith CH, Graham N, Lilge L, Burnie S, White R. "Low Level Laser Therapy (LLLT) for Neck Pain: A Systematic Review and Meta-Regression." *Open Orthop J.* (2013) Sep 20;7:396-419. doi: 10.2174/1874325001307010396. eCollection 2013.

Iannitti T1, Fistetto G, Esposito A, Rottigni V, Palmieri B. "Pulsed electromagnetic field therapy for management of osteoarthritis-related pain, stiffness and physical function: clinical experience in the elderly." *Clin Interv Aging.* (2013);8:1289-93. doi: 10.2147/CIA.S35926. Epub 2013 Sep 26.

Institute of Medicine Report from the Committee on Advancing Pain Research, Care, and Education: Relieving Pain in America, A Blueprint for Transforming Prevention, Care, Education and Research. *The National Academies Press* (2011). *books.nap.edu/openbook. php?record_id=13172&page=1.*

Lipo-Spheric GSH: *livonlabs.com*

Low level lasers: *lucklaser.com*

NutraMedix Burbur Detox, Parsley Detox and Pinella: *NutraMedix.com*

Oke KI1, Umebese PF2. "Evaluation of the efficacy of pulsed electromagnetic therapy in the treatment of back pain: a randomized controlled trial in a tertiary hospital in Nigeria." *West Indian Med J.*(2013 Mar);62(3):205-9

Omar AS1, Awadalla MA, El-Latif MA. "Evaluation of pulsed electromagnetic field therapy in the management of patients with discogenic lumbar radiculopathy." *Int J Rheum Dis.* (2012 Oct);15(5):e101-8. doi: 10.1111/j.1756-185X.2012.01745.x.

Pereira, T. et al. « Efficacy of red and infrared lasers in treatment of temporomandibular disorders-a double-blind, randomized, parallel clinical trial." *Cranio.* (2014 Jan);32(1):51-6.

ReadiSorb: *readisorb.com*

Soleimanpour H1, Gahramani K, Taheri R, Golzari SE, Safari S, Esfanjani RM, Iranpour A. "The effect of low-level laser therapy on knee osteoarthritis: prospective, descriptive study." *Lasers Med Sci.* (2014 Apr 15).

Vickers, A. et al. "Acupuncture for chronic pain. Individual patient data meta-analysis." (2012, Oct.) *JAMA Internal Medicine.* Oct 22, 2012, Vol 172, No. 19 *archinte.jamanetwork.com/article.aspx?articleid=1357513*

CHAPTERS 23-26

Bioenergetic Treatments for Insomnia—Neurofeedback, Light and Sound Machines, Homeopathy, Energetic Remedies, Biomat, PEMF, Alpha-Stim Devices

Alpha-Stim devices: *alpha-stim.com*

Babuna, Amantilla: *NutraMedix.com*

Biomat: *Biomat.com*

Curtin, D. "Sleep Problems." *British Homeopathic Association.* Retrieved on April 14, 2014 from: *britishhomeopathic.org/bha-charity/how-we-can-help/conditions-a-z/sleep-problems/*

Hammer BU1, Colbert AP, Brown KA, Ilioi EC. "Neurofeedback for insomnia: a pilot study of Z-score SMR and individualized protocols." *Appl Psychophysiol Biofeedback.* (2011 Dec);36(4):251-64. doi: 10.1007/s10484-011-9165-y.

Hauri PJ, Percy L, Hellekson C, Hartmann E, Russ D. "The treatment of psychophysiologic insomnia with biofeedback: a replication study." *Biofeedback Self Regul.* (1982 Jun);7(2):223-35.

iMRS: *IMRS. Com* (Mediconsult) *imrs.com/en/*

Sound-Light Machines: *ToolsForWellness.com*

Walker, J., Lawson, R., Koslowski, G. "Current Status of QEEG and Neurofeedback in the Treatment of Clinical Depression." *Neurotherapy Center of Dallas clearmindcenter.com/Research/Bipolar/Depression-Walker_2006.pdf*

Chapters 27-31

Bioenergetic Treatments for Depression—Neurofeedback, EVOX, EFT, REMAP, EMDR, etc.

Bisson JI1, Roberts NP, Andrew M, Cooper R, Lewis C. "Psychological therapies for chronic post-traumatic stress disorder (PTSD) in adults." Cochrane Database Syst Rev. (2013 Dec 13);12:CD003388. doi: 10.1002/14651858.CD003388.pub4.

Church D1, Yount G, Brooks AJ. "The effect of emotional freedom techniques on stress biochemistry: a randomized controlled trial." *J Nerv Ment Dis.* (2012 Oct);200(10):891-6. doi: 10.1097/NMD.0b013e31826b9fc1.

EFT Practitioners. *Association for Comprehensive Energy Psychology.* Retrieved on April 20, 2014 from: *energypsych.site-ym.com/search/custom.asp?id=1721*

Emotional Freedom Technique: *Emofree.com*

EMDR Institute: *EMDR.com*

EMDR Therapists. *EMDR International Association.* Retrieved on April 20, 2014 from: *emdria.org/displaycommon. cfm?an=1&subarticlenbr=235*

EVOX Therapy: *ZYTO.com/evox.html*

"Lack Energy? Maybe It's Your Magnesium Level." *Agricultural Research* (2004, May).

Lee, C.W., & Cuijpers, P. "A meta-analysis of the contribution of eye movements in processing emotional memories." *Journal of Behavior Therapy & Experimental Psychiatry,* (2013) 44, 231-239.

Lehman, K. "EMDR and Theophostic: FAQ's and Common Misunderstandings." Retrieved on April 10, 2014 from: *kclehman.com/download. php?doc=29*

"Mood Disorders." *National Institute of Mental health. nimh.nih.gov/ health/publications/the-numbers-count-mental-disorders-in-america/ index.shtml*

REMAP Therapy: *remapinstitute.org*

Stapleton P1, Church D, Sheldon T, Porter B, Carlopio C. "Depression symptoms improve after successful weight loss with emotional freedom techniques." *ISRN Psychiatry.* 2013 Jul 28;2013:573532. doi: 10.1155/2013/573532. eCollection 2013.

CHAPTERS 32-34

Bioenergetic Treatments for Anxiety—Homeopathy, Homotoxicology, Bach Flower Remedies, Rubimed, Reflexology, etc.

Clear Mind Center research studies: *clearmindcenter.com/Research/ Bipolar/Depression-Walker_2006.pdf*

Guide to the Remedies. *The Bach Centre: bachcentre.com/centre/remedies. htm*

Heel Products: *Heel.com*

Homeopathic Academy of Naturopathic Physicians. Retrieved on April 20, 2014 from: *hanp.net/general/directory*

Introduction to Homotoxicology. International Academy of Homotoxicology. (2007). Retrieved on April 10, 2014 from: *iah-online.com/cms/ docs/doc26605.pdf*

National Center for Homeopathy: *homeopathycenter.org*

Oliva i Segura M. "Emotional support and Bach Flower Therapy." *Rev Enferm.* (2009 Oct);32(10):16-9.

Pekana Products: *Pekana.com*

Rubimed Therapy: *rubimed.com*

The Original Bach Flower Remedies. Retrieved on April 12, 2014 from: *bachflower.com/what-is-anxiety-what-causes-anxiety/*

What is homeopathy? *The Society of Homeopaths*. Retrieved on April 14, 2014 from: *homeopathy-soh.org/about-homeopathy/what-is-homeopathy/*

Wong, C. Reflexology. *About.com*. Retrieved on April 17, 2014 from: *altmedicine.about.com/od/therapiesfromrtoz/a/Reflexology.htm-*

W. Lee Cowden, MD, MD(H)

W. Lee Cowden, MD, MD(H), is a U.S. board-certified cardiologist and internist internationally renowned and recognized for his knowledge and skill in practicing and teaching integrative medicine.

He is Chairman of the Scientific Advisory Board and Academy Professor for the Academy of Comprehensive Integrative Medicine (ACIM). ACIM is dedicated to shifting the healthcare paradigm toward wellness by training and supporting practitioners in a variety of holistic health disciplines; conducting research, and implementing therapeutic innovations to create a new global wellness care community.

Dr. Cowden has pioneered successful treatments for a myriad of diseases, including chronic fatigue syndrome, cancer, autism, fibromyalgia, heart disease, Lyme disease, and others.

In addition to treating thousands of patients, Dr. Cowden travels and teaches integrative medicine nationally and internationally in countries such as Mexico, Brazil, Peru, Guatemala, Germany, the Czech Republic, Japan, China, Taiwan, England, the Netherlands, Austria, Australia, Norway, Curaçao, the Dominican Republic, Singapore and Malaysia. He is also a member of the Lyme and Autism Foundation scientific advisory board.

Dr. Cowden is the author or co-author of many publications, including the following books:

Insights into Lyme Disease Treatment (2009)

Longevity, An Alternative Medicine Definitive Guide (2001)

Cancer Diagnosis: What to Do Next (2000)

The best-selling *An Alternative Medicine Definitive Guide to Cancer* (1997).

Although Dr. Cowden was initially trained in traditional, allopathic medicine early on in his career, he realized that this type of medicine often not only didn't heal his patients, but frequently failed to bring them to a place of wellness and ultimate wholeness so that their illnesses wouldn't recur. With this realization, he undertook a program to expand his knowledge, experience and medical practice to include natural, non-toxic, holistic solutions for wellness.

More than a holistic physician, Dr. Cowden is also a sensitive educator who teaches lifestyle, emotional and spiritual strategies for living well so that his patients can go beyond wellness to wholeness—in body, mind and spirit.

More information about Dr. Cowden and his work can be found on the Academy of Comprehensive Integrative Medicine website: *ACIMConnect.com.*

Connie Strasheim

Connie Strasheim is a medical researcher and writer who has experienced the hardships of chronic illness firsthand through her near decade-long battle with Lyme disease and chronic fatigue syndrome.

Besides coauthoring the books in this series, she is the author of five books on holistic treatments for disease. They include:

The best-selling *Insights into Lyme Disease Treatment: Thirteen Lyme-Literate Health Care Practitioners Share Their Healing Strategies* (2009)

Beyond Lyme Disease: Healing The Underlying Causes of Chronic Illness in People with Borreliosis and Co-Infections (2012)

Defeat Cancer: 15 Doctors of Integrative and Naturopathic Medicine Tell You How (2010)

Healing Chronic Illness: By His Spirit, Through His Resources
(2010)

The Lyme Disease Survival Guide: Physical, Lifestyle and Emotional Strategies for Healing (2008).

Through her battle with severe chronic illness, Connie has learned that attaining wellness isn't just about eliminating infections, detoxifying the body or balancing the hormones—it's about addressing all the factors that caused the body to break down in the first place. These include all environmental, psycho-emotional, lifestyle and spiritual issues that cause or contribute to damage, discontent and—ultimately—"dis-ease" in the body, mind and spirit.

She has also learned, through her experience and research, that in order to be well—never mind being whole—in today's world fraught with stress and toxicity, many tools are required. In this book series, *The Journey to Wellness,* she and Dr. Cowden share some of these tools.

More information about Connie's work can be found on her website: *ConnieStrasheim.com.*

ACIM Press The Journey to Wellness Book Series

Did you know that toxins are a primary cause of most chronic and degenerative diseases today, such as chronic fatigue syndrome, Alzheimers, fibromyalgia, heart disease, Parkinson's, irritable bowel syndrome, and cancer? Fortunately, you can heal from your current health condition or simply optimize your health by removing these toxins from your home and body. In *Create a Toxin-Free Body and Home...Starting Today,* W. Lee Cowden, MD and Connie Strasheim tell you how!

First, the authors describe how to identify hidden, dangerous environmental toxins that are found in most homes, as well as in the air, food and water supply. They then describe ways to remove these toxins from the body, using everything from do-it-yourself, easy hands-on manual therapies, to doctor-assisted chelation, oral supplements, and more.

ACIM
The Journey to Wellness Book Series

Create a Toxin-Free Body & Home Starting Today

W. Lee Cowden, MD, MD(H)
Connie Strasheim

Finally, they teach you how to make healthy lifestyle choices to avoid re-exposure to toxins and to maintain your health and well-being. For more information, visit: *ACIMConnect.com.*

ACIM Press

Most diet books today focus on a one-size-fits-all approach to food selection. In *Foods that Fit a Unique You*, authors W. Lee Cowden, MD and Connie Strasheim prove that no two people have the same biochemistry and needs, and that one-size-fit-all food plans are therefore inadequate for determining what you need to eat for optimal health, fitness and weight maintenance.

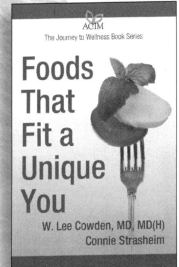

In *Foods that Fit a Unique You*, the authors teach you how to identify truly healthy foods, and look and feel your best, by taking into account six individual factors, including:

- Your body's pH
- Your food allergies
- Your metabolic type
- Your gastrointestinal function
- Foods that clump your red blood cells together
- Your current health condition

In *Foods that Fit a Unique You*, the authors provide general guidelines on how to identify and choose healthy foods, and then teach you how to find the foods that will best fit your unique body, based on the above factors.

They then show you how to avoid food allergens, optimize your digestion and heal your gastrointestinal tract, so that you can get the most out of your meals. For more information, visit: *ACIMConnect.com*.

ACIM Press

Conventional medicine has limited tools for identifying and treating the cause of common, but frequently elusive symptoms, such as fatigue, pain, insomnia, depression and anxiety. Vitamins, herbs and drugs, as well as conventional healing tools, such as surgery, counseling, chiropractic care and physical therapy, often fail to help people to heal from these conditions.

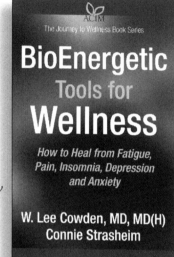

Fortunately, bioenergetic medicine can provide gentle, safe and effective healing solutions when other methods fail. In *BioEnergetic Wellness Tools: How to Heal from Fatigue, Pain, Insomnia, Depression, and Anxiety*, authors W. Lee Cowden, MD and Connie Strasheim explain the advantages of bioenergetic medicine over other types of healing modalities.

They then share the bioenergetic tools that they have found to be most effective for healing the body from five often difficult-to-treat conditions, including fatigue, pain, insomnia, depression and anxiety. These tools range from inexpensive and gentle homeopathic and energetically-imprinted remedies, to powerful energetic devices, do-it-yourself hands-on healing techniques, and diagnostic devices that help to detect imbalances and problems in the body.

Discover the tools that can help you to recover from conditions that conventional medicine has failed to treat! For more information, visit: *ACIMConnect.com*.

Made in the USA
San Bernardino, CA
21 June 2019